BEFORE THE AGE OF MIRACLES

William Victor Johnston M.D.

BEFORE THE AGE OF MIRACLES

Memoirs of a Country Doctor

Foreword by Dr. E. K. Lyon

Paul S. Eriksson, Inc.
New York, N.Y.

First published in Canada
by
Fitzhenry & Whiteside, Limited,
Toronto, Ont.

and by

Paul S. Eriksson, Inc.,
New York, N.Y.

ISBN 0-8397-1023-2

Printed and bound in Canada by
the T. H. Best Printing Company Limited

Contents

Acknowledgements

I am grateful to a considerable company of persons who provided information, guidance and encouragement: Dr. John Hamilton, Vice-President of Health Sciences, University of Toronto Medical School; Mrs. Elizabeth Kalashnikoff, former editor of Harper & Row, for advice concerning arrangements of text and format; Mr. C. J. Eustace, publishers' consultant and author, Toronto, Ontario; and Mr. Earl Damude, Editor, *Medical Post,* Maclean-Hunter Ltd. For information about certain diseases and their treatment, I am indebted to: Dr. William W. Wigle, President, Pharmaceutical Manufacturers Association of Canada; Dr. Kenneth Ferguson, Director, Connaught Medical Research Laboratories; Dr. Eddie O'Brian, former Vice-President, Ontario Tuberculosis and Respiratory Disease Association; Mr. Howard I. Murray, former Vice-President of J. F. Hartz Co. Ltd.; Dr. H. Hutchins, Medical Director, G. D. Searle & Company; Dr. Milo Tyndel, Psychiatrist, Toronto; and Professor George H. V. Lucas, formerly Professor of Pharmacology, University of Toronto. For consultation on children's diseases, I would like to thank Dr. Nelles Silverthorne; Dr. Harry Bain; Dr. A. W. Farmer; Dr. Edward Morgan; and family doctors: Dr. E. K. Lyon, Leamington, Ontario; Dr. Murray M. Fisher, Gravenhurst, Ontario; Dr. George E. Case, Newmarket, Ontario; Dr. Gilbert Parker, Toronto, Ontario; Dr. R. E. Ives, Stayner, Ontario; Dr. M. H. Corrin, Lucknow, Ontario. A grant of $1,500 from the Canada Council in 1969 enabled me to begin this work.

Foreword

Much has been written of the clinical and scientific triumphs of the nineteen twenties and thirties but very little has been recorded of the work of the country family doctor of that time.

Deprived of the modern and sophisticated diagnostic methods of today, the country doctor had to depend on inspection, palpation, percussion and auscultation, spiced with a large measure of his God-given senses, in order to arrive at a diagnosis and management of his patient.

Treatment was often empiric and largely depended on preserving the patient's natural body resources for its success.

Dr. William Victor Johnston was born in Huron County, Ontario, just prior to the turn of the century. His boyhood was spent in a rural setting. After education in the local schools he attended Victoria College, in Toronto, where he received his B.A. degree. He was then attracted to the profession of medicine and received his M.D. degree from Toronto in 1923. In 1924 he began practice in Lucknow, Ontario, a small village not far from the place of his birth. Here he spent the next thirty years of his life caring for the illnesses of the people in the village and surrounding country.

Dr. Johnston's account of his concern, not only for his patients' physical complaints, but his deep interest in their worries and frustrations, typifies those qualities we would all like to find in our own family physician.

In spite of the difficulties of practicing in a rural area, deep in the snow belt of Ontario, during an economic depression, raising and educating a family, Dr. Johnston found time to take short postgraduate courses to improve his knowledge. He found time to give of himself to the business of his profession and in 1949 became President of the Ontario Medical Association and filled this office with distinction.

During this period of his life Dr. Johnston became firmly convinced that, if the family physician was to fulfill his proper place in the medical world, opportunities and incentives must be provided for continuing medical education. He spent many hours and days away from his home, family and practice, promoting his concept. In 1954 he saw the beginning of his dream come true when the College of Family Physicians of Canada was formed. It was a logical sequence that he should be the choice of that body to become its first Executive Director—a position he held from 1954 until his retirement in 1965. This new position occupied him on a full time basis and it was with some regret that he gave up his rural practice and his close contacts with patients.

During his tenure of office as the Executive Director he saw the College grow from a few members to its present state as a countrywide entity, dedicated to the advancement of knowledge of the family physician of Canada.

Since retirement Dr. Johnston has continued his interest in his profession and the welfare of mankind, serving with the Alcoholism and Drug Addiction Research Foundation.

In recognition of his untiring efforts on behalf of his colleagues in family practice and the people they serve, Dr. Johnston has received many honors. He is a life member of the Ontario Medical Association, a senior member of the Canadian Medical Association, an honorary Fellow of the Colleges of General Practice of Great Britain and Australia, and holds a Fellowship of the College of Family Physicians of Canada. The University of Western Ontario honored him with the degree of LL.D. (Honoris Causa) in 1966.

Perhaps the greatest recognition of his service to his profession has been conferred on him by the College of Family Physicians for which he has done so much. In 1965 the College struck the William Victor Johnston Medal of Honor, to be awarded annually to an outstanding member of the College, and accompanying that, established the William Victor Johnston Oration, to be given by a speaker on invitation at its annual assembly.

In these modern days when the "prophets" of the future tell us that the family physician may be replaced by the computer, Dr. Johnston's memoirs of a country family doctor, recounting experiences in family practice *Before the Age of Miracles* should encourage the modern day family physician, with his improved diagnostic and therapeutic tools, to maintain his rightful rôle in the practice of medicine as physician, counsellor, confidant, and friend of the people he serves.

E. K. Lyon, M.D.
Medical Centre, Leamington, Ontario.

To my children
Katherine, Mary, Bruce and Nancy

Prologue

What is gone by should perhaps remain behind. Satchel Page, the Negro baseball pitcher and sage, is reported to have said, "Never look back, something might be gaining on you." Certainly today's youth, our leaders of tomorrow, are impatient with the accomplishments of their seniors and care little what an old man is thinking. Yet there is another view possible. Dr. Christiaan N. Barnard, in his teaching, stresses that "the longer we look backward, the further we can look forward." In the current climate of rapid change all about us the medical profession, and particularly that part engaged in general practice, is carefully reassessing its services with the hope it can retain the good and discard the bad. But in order to decide which is which much of the past must be recalled and evaluated.

I was a general practitioner for thirty years—1924-1954—in Lucknow, Ontario, a village on the boundary line between the counties of Huron and Bruce in the western part of southern Ontario, which had a scant population of one thousand souls. Another two thousand in the surrounding area were dependent upon the services I and a few colleagues could provide. In looking back, I think of myself as a family doctor, a term I prefer to "general practitioner" and "general physician" though I use them all interchangeably.

There are many reasons for this preference and one of them is especially worth stressing. General practitioners in Canada, under the leadership of their college (College of Family Physicians), for the past few years have been calling themselves family physicians. This is much more than a mere change of name. To a degree never attempted before they are probing the dynamics of the family, the natural unit of our society. Already this research, aided particularly by psychiatrists, is yielding an amazing amount of new information. Furthermore, through changes in the curricula of medical schools, preparation for the practice of family medicine is becoming as long and as arduous as training for the traditional specialists. There is a concerted effort to make a community family doctor a specialist family doctor in his own right.

The suggestion for this book came from Dr. John Hamilton, Vice-President of Health Sciences of the University of Toronto Medical School, who has felt the need for an accurate recording of the work of practicing doctors of my period. Though much has been written about medical associations, hospitals and organizations of the era—such as the Neurological Institute of Montreal and the Connaught Medical Research Laboratories in Toronto—relatively little has been recorded of what the doctors in the field were doing, in offices, homes and hospitals. Such a meticulous reporting, Dr. Hamilton said, might even serve as source material for future medical students. As a final bit of advice he added, "Many books about general practitioners are chiefly chronicles or collections of anecdotes. I am asking for a book about medicine."

So it was that this narrative of my life and the life of my time as a doctor came to be written. It is not intended as an autobiography. If its early chapters seem to be too much about myself, the reader is reminded that I am trying to present the origins and motivations of a typical Canadian practitioner of my period with his typical weaknesses, strengths, faults and virtues—nothing more. The later chapters suggest the learning process by which I achieved a personal point of view, with case histories for illustration. The book is about the interchange between a doctor and his patients in which the doctor sometimes received more than he gave. If it accomplishes its intention, it will make clear how the doctor of thirty years ago compensated for his lack of scientific knowledge by his sympathetic understanding of the patient and by his intimate knowledge of the patient's family. He drew heavily on his treasure of facts about what stressed certain persons and what liberated them. In doing so, physicians of my time gave a personalized service which was uniquely effective for the reason that they were working from a position of great strength—namely, that their patients trusted them.

It should be kept in mind that the period of which I write saw a great revolution in medicine as in other fields. Socially, in the 1920's we were living in an economic atmosphere vastly different from that of today. A haircut and shave was fifty cents, milk ten cents a quart, and gasoline was about the same price as today if you remember that there was no government tax then. The Dominion Bureau of Statistics tells me that a dollar in 1924 has shrunk in value to 47½ cents today. This can be stated in another way: a dollar then would purchase what today costs about $2.10. In spite of what many say, since 1920 the incomes of most people have increased faster than expenses and this, along with health insurance, has substantially increased the health resources available to the ailing.

I started medical practice shortly before there was insulin for the diabetic or liver extract for pernicious anemia and long before any of the antibiotics. We had no "stopper" or "starter" drugs—the so-called mood-altering pills which can pep you up and calm you down, and no pills to control fertility. There were few aids for the physically handicapped and mentally retarded. Most babies were born in the homes and some major surgery was done there.

In the 1920's, the anemias of my patients were often of the pernicious type. Infections lasted a long time and youth faded fast for those who survived childhood. Many people aged early with wheezing chests and creaking joints, yet through it all they dearly loved pleasure and were remarkably resilient in bouncing back from injury and sickness.

Family medicine has advanced light years from the horse-and-buggy days of the traditional general practitioner. The horse died and the buggy crumbled into dust when the cool voice of science flooded into family medicine, at the same time that it worked revolutionary changes in transportation.

In my day, a rural and small-town doctor like myself was interviewing each week from Sunday to Sunday about two hundred people. This is at a rate of ten thousand a year. He met all the emotions from fright to lust. The average rural doctor had about twenty-five deaths a year and about twice as many births. He dealt with countless colds, much indigestion, many anemias, chronic bronchitis, and urinary infections. He was presented with an occasional suicide and abortion, a little madness, and much personal misery from worry and anxiety.

This and more is the substance of my story as it attempts to answer such questions as these: What did the old-time family doctors, their consultants and helpers do for the sick and injured under their care? What did the patients themselves do for their doctors? What therapeutic skills did the doctors master when by today's standards their therapeutic arsenal was so scant? How did the doctors grapple with the growing stockpile of new drugs, facilities and techniques? Having in mind that in any age accurate diagnosis is the hallmark of quality medical care, how did the physicians of my day measure up in this regard? How did the doctors live with the continuous demands for their services when, as now, sickness had no hours and death no holiday and transportation was neither swift nor sure?

My experience may supply some helpful answers. I hope so.

I. In the Beginning . . . Family and Schooling

I have always been a bit envious of those who have had a "call" or sense of mission in life. God's hand on their shoulder seems to make them more courageous and possibly more successful than the rest of us. Though many doctors knew in their youth what they wanted to be, I am sure that for many others considerations apart from dedication influenced their choice. In my own case, I just drifted into medicine.

I was fourteen years old when I finished public school, squeaking through the so-called entrance examinations with ten marks over the 380-point minimum. Father had his own way of thinking about his children's education. He kept me on the farm the following two years. Then one September day he casually asked, "Son, would you like to go back to school?"

"Yes, I think so."

"What would you like to study?"

"I don't know."

"All right. You can start in Lucknow High School next week and you can go as long as you wish, providing you pass each year. But remember, if you fail a year you will be back on the farm."

There was no discussion whatever about where education might lead me or any advantage it might bring. His only interest was: Would I like it? Could I pass? I welcomed the opportunity. Though I was reared on a farm and was expected to handle horses, I had very little interest in animals. My brother knew every horse on the road, whereas I couldn't identify even those of the nearest neighbors.

Father kept his word about schooling, with no questioning, for eleven years while I progressed from Lucknow and Wingham high schools to Victoria College for a B.A., and then to medical school in Toronto. Perhaps I should explain that Father had two farms of four hundred or so acres. Every spring he imported a sawmill to saw 120,000 square feet of lumber. From this supplementary income came some of the money for my education.

Early, I discovered that I had a good memory. I could memorize whole blocks of history, Latin, poems, and mathematics. A friend had successfully taken grades XII and XIII with some seventeen subjects in one year and dared me to do the same. I accomplished this, although it wasn't a very distinguished feat as I did nothing but study, with little or no time off for social life or sports. For several reasons, I decided I had done these two years too hurriedly and I voluntarily took another year to repeat them. The second time around I received an Edward Blake Scholarship. It was small, only $45 annually for three years, but it enticed me into entering Victoria College, which was a Methodist church school until it joined with others to form Toronto University.

A friend studying for the Presbyterian ministry persuaded me to register as a student for the Methodist ministry at Victoria, but two weeks of Greek and Hebrew were enough for me. From long hours of French and Latin in high school I was convinced that I had no further interest in languages, so I shifted to a science course—biology and physics. On completion I could qualify to become a high school science teacher or enter third-year medical course.

All went smoothly until the fourth year, when I found myself memorizing difficult equations because I was unable to think them through. For example, I learned by rote how to estimate the speed of gas molecules under particular temperatures and pressures. It became obvious to me that it would never do for a high school teacher to be unable to reason its problems, so I abandoned this field as a possible vocation and entered the third-year class of medicine.

My difficulty in settling on a life work taught me never to hurry my four children into choosing a vocation. I insisted that there must be a place for them to test themselves by trial and error if opportunity offered.

I looked upon high school and university examinations as contests without many rules and worked out two little tricks that served to ease me past the examiners. First, I studied every evening, every weekend including Sunday and every holiday, guided by a precise program: one hour for subject A, then a half hour for subject B, and so on, often alternating the dull and interesting subjects. I left nothing in the choice of subject to guesswork. Second, as part of my preparation for the annual spring examinations, I went home immediately before them for a week's holiday to forget about schooling and to eat, sleep, and work on the farm. It took all my courage to try this but once tried, it became an annual pattern.

I had promised Father to help him each summer on the farm where he was always short-handed. This meant that I couldn't work in hospitals during the holidays as many of my classmates were doing. On a couple of occasions this commitment interfered with attractive offers of special experience. Once the late Professor Walker of the Biology Department of Toronto University invited me to spend a summer at the famous Woods Hole marine biological station on Cape Cod. Another time the late Dr. Velyien Henderson, Professor of Pharmacology of the Toronto Medical School, asked me to analyze, under his supervision during a summer holiday, one of the numerous false skin cancer cures rife in Ontario. I knew that one of these so-called remedies was in demand in my home county of Bruce because my grandmother had applied the black messy ointment to an arm cancer. Though it burned her skin fiercely, it didn't save her life. Dr. Henderson guessed that the key ingredient in these quack cures was arsenic and he wanted to test this surmise. That I couldn't accept either of these offers deprived me of valuable experience, I am sure. How valuable, it is difficult to estimate.

Although the study of medicine was intensely interesting, it didn't smother all my other interests. The summer preceding my last year of medical school, rather than intern in a hospital, I joined Frontier College. Right or wrong, I felt I needed a change from the medical atmosphere.

Since 1900, long before anyone dreamed of a Company of Young Canadians or an American Peace Corps, Frontier College had been sending university students to logging camps, to work gangs on roads, railways, etc., as worker-teachers. The students were expected to live on the money they earned as members of the work force but they were paid extra for teaching the workmen whatever they wished to study in off-hours.

I was assigned to a gang on the rugged railroad stretch in the Rockies between Calgary and Field. The workmen were mostly Russians with a scattering of Scandinavians, Italians, and English. In the evenings I read Dickens' *Little Dorrit* with a Norwegian lad who was taking three years to work his way around the world in lieu of a university education, and at the moment was learning English. Occasionally I joined four Scots who were avid students of Karl Marx's *Das Kapital*. The Russians, without exception, preferred instruction in mathematics.

I have never regretted this social experiment, which taught me the ways of workmen and took me tramping about the mountains on weekends and holidays with a knapsack on my back. That summer was probably the best holiday I ever had.

Frontier College still exists and is quite active throughout Canada, with a unit in each province. I am told that the Ontario division has an annual budget of $120,000 from the provincial government and in 1969 sent out 24 students who contacted more than 300,000 workmen and gave instruction to 1,848.

Why did I choose general practice rather than one of the specialties? This is not an easy question to answer. I know that I had a subconscious wish to deal with all types of people in the full commitment of their lives. Never could I see myself listening all day with a stethoscope to chest sounds, or looking down throats, or up rectums. Other specialized fields which I felt were easier than general practice struck me as equally boring. I am thinking particularly of skin specialists, whose patients rarely die, and X-ray experts, whose expensive equipment is usually owned by clinics or hospitals and who seem to lead leisurely lives interpreting films while sitting in comfortable chairs. (This is no doubt an over-simplification.) Major surgery I considered beyond my capabilities, believing that it called for a particular temperament and aptitudes I didn't have. Unquestionably, the enormous demand for family doctor services helped to influence my choice. About eighty-five percent of human ills are common in nature and respond to direct measures, making it of some importance to be proficient in many ailments. Then as now, I considered general practice one of the most difficult fields of medicine because a competent general practitioner must be one of the most expert diagnosticians. He not only must know when he can help but, what is just as important, he must be quick to recognize a situation that is beyond him and refer such a seriously ill patient to more expert care than he can give.

All of this can be true and still not explain fully why I chose as I did. Perhaps—who knows?—my ancestors and my particular upbringing may have had much to do with it.

My father, Albert E. Johnston, was an Irishman descended from lowland Scots transported to Ireland by Cromwell. They came from one of the three robber border clans, the Scotts, Douglases, and Johnstons, who were notorious as raiders of their neighbors for fun and profit.

Mother, born Honor Perkins, was Devonshire English, her forebears Flemish weavers who fled to England to escape religious persecution.

The two were married in Ontario in 1894 and I was born May 9, 1897. Dr. Thomas Case, of the hamlet of Dungannon, four miles distant, brought me into the world, for which services Father paid him seven dollars. I have it on good authority that Dr. Case never grossed as much as five thousand dollars in any year of fifty years' practice.

Many years later Mother confided that my birth was a disappointment. The year 1897 was that of Queen Victoria's Jubilee and she had prayed for a girl to be named Victoria. Since I was not that kind of baby, she just shortened the name to Victor.

A brother preceded me by a year. At two months he was left in the care of a neighbor while my parents went to the village to shop. He was dead when they returned, my father believed from an unaccustomed feeding of bread and milk. This is possible. I have seen a breastfed baby seriously disturbed by such a feeding but have not known one to die of it. Only once did I ever hear this brother mentioned. There were no pictures—nothing to indicate that he had ever lived. A brother and two sisters followed my birth.

My conscious life began with a barn raising. Freud somewhere says that we do not recall events earlier than five years, yet I have heard people say their memory carries them back to two years and even earlier. At the time of this barn raising I was four years old.

Barn raising and chopping bees were the kind of cooperative activities on which this country was built in the early days when common difficulties brought families together. I recall vividly the details of that barn raising. It was a mass onslaught of one hundred or more neighbors. In one afternoon they put together the beam framework of a sixty-by-eighty foot building. Once this framework was up, the work could be finished at a leisurely pace by a small crew of professional carpenters. The day ended with a rousing contest between two teams chosen by captains. Each team undertook to put up the rafter framework of half the roof, racing to be the first to finish. With the noisy shouting of orders, and men climbing wildly over the framework as they tossed pieces of lumber about with abandon, it was a miracle no one was injured. The winning team eventually swung nimbly to the ground, privileged to be the first to sample the food from rows of heavily laden tables under the orchard apple trees. And what a spread! Roast chicken and roast beef, home-made bread and rolls, dozens of cakes and pies, jugs of milk, buttermilk, and lemonade. There may have been some apple cider or a stronger beverage hidden somewhere about, but I didn't see any.

My parents were Methodists and lived this faith. Newspapers were put away Saturday evening and no work was done on Sunday except to look after the stock—not even shoes were shined. Playing cards were forbidden in the house, although we had Lost Heir and Dominoes. A small library of several dozen volumes included Carlisle's *History of the French Revolution*, a history of the South African war, *Robinson Crusoe*, and a series of Henty's adventure stories. Also, there was Milton's *Paradise Lost*, which I remember chiefly because to me this epic of the fight between good and evil was quite uninteresting.

Every day after breakfast and before starting work Father would read a chapter from the Bible followed by prayer. This occurred regardless of who was working for us or visiting, or how busy we were. It seemed to give Father strength to meet the bustle and the annoyances of the day. On Sunday mornings we all went to Donnybrook church three miles distant—in a buggy in summer and by cutter in winter. The service was invariably followed by a short period when the adults met in groups to give testimony about their progress in the Christian faith. Father led one of these groups.

Sunday afternoons were usually very dull for me and I acquired the habit of using this part of the week for wandering about the countryside. In this way I became interested in the flora of the meadows, woods and bogs. With the aid of H. B. Spotton's descriptive catalogue of flowers, plants and grasses, I was able to identify most of them and I found after a few trials that I could make quite presentable pencil drawings of what I observed. As with painting and other skills, we don't know what we can do until we try.

Apart from Sundays, every day in summer was a work day except for three special occasions. On July 12th Father always took the family to the nearest "Orange Walk," though he was never an Orangeman. He disliked the dogma of the order. The church picnic in a beech and maple grove on the banks of the Maitland River also called for a holiday, as did the Fall Fair of the nearby village of Dungannon.

Understandably, there was never a drop of whiskey in a Methodist household but Father, bless him, was no zealot. He never preached about his manner of living—he just lived it. The only instruction he ever gave my brother and me about alcohol was, "If you don't drink or smoke before you are twenty-one I will give each of you a gold watch. After that you may do as you please." We observed his directive, but he forgot about the watch. I am sure this was merely an oversight.

Father always raised a field of barley that was used to fatten the hogs. It was many years later when I learned why he wouldn't sell the barley; he figured it would find its way into beer.

One of his dictums was: "Don't make up your mind about religion until you are a grown man." I recall riding home with him on a load of hay from a secondary farm he had two miles away. It was during the summer holidays following my second year at Victoria. I had entered a new world of wonders and revelation and I undertook to tell him about the probable evolution of mankind from lower creatures over millenia of years and the likelihood that it all may not have started with Adam and Eve in the Garden of Eden. Dad just listened. This was an embarrassment, as I had to keep talking and probably said more than I intended. Finally, on arrival at the home barn, he observed quietly, "Son, never take an old man's religion away from him until you have something better to put in its place." That ended for a long time any attempt to lecture him on what to believe.

For some reason I was always closer to my father than to Mother. As you may guess, Father was the dominant partner. Mother was a very different type of person. She was all kindness and sweetness, forever scrubbing, cleaning, cooking and mending. The only public meetings she attended were church socials and quilting bees. I never heard a serious argument between my parents, though Mother did complain at times of too little money. She loved to spend money, and I am sure she felt she never had enough. The rather meager weekly egg-and-butter money was hers and each year around the tenth of December was a gala day when she received the bonanza of her turkey proceeds.

Each year we carefully nurtured to maturity a hundred turkeys. I recall how in the fall they began roosting at night in the apple orchard about the time the autumn winds started tearing off the dead leaves. On late November evenings it was a thrilling sight to see those hundred large birds swaying on the topmost limbs of the sixty-foot-high Spy trees, all facing the wind. The black turkeys of that day were wilder and nobler birds than the white ones we raise today. On the sudden whim of a leader, they would sometimes all fly five hundred yards or so to another feeding ground.

About a hundred plucked turkeys went to the storekeeper on December 10th when Mother exchanged them for winter clothing, Christmas presents and always a crate of California oranges. It was a perfect day if she didn't have a nickel left when it was over. May the Lord bless her!

There was very little serious illness in the family. Every few weeks the children got a dose of castor oil and we vied with each other in pretending how much we liked it. Each spring we got some sulphur and black strap molasses. I don't know what the sulphur did for us, but the molasses was rich in iron in an easily assimilated form. Even today, at some drug stores, a mixture of sulphur, molasses, and cream of tartar can be obtained.

Dental services were very limited. For an aching tooth or one with a large cavity, I was taken to a Dr. Bice in Dungannon. He never filled a tooth, he just pulled it out. No anaesthetic—one jerk which would almost lift me off the chair and the tooth was in his hand. As a result, I didn't have a tooth filled until I was in my late twenties and it is little wonder that I began to use false teeth in my early fifties.

It was out of such a background—not unique but made up of countless familiar elements—that I emerged. When I finished medical school in 1923 my father told me that I owed him nothing. In explanation, he said that he had willed everything he had to Mother during her lifetime; after that my brother and two sisters would inherit. My education was my share of his patrimony. With a twinkle in his eye he added that he hoped I would look after him should he ever require medical attention.

. . . Teachers

For the mental furniture with which I started my career, I am indebted to the dedicated physicians who were my teachers. I owe them everything, and I say this without reservation.

It was Easter 1923 when I found myself in the hamlet of Sprucedale deep in the Muskoka region of northern Ontario. I was looking forward to graduation in medicine two months later and as a respite from study I went to Sprucedale to help an elderly physician, Dr. George Richardson, for two weeks. I arrived there nearly frozen after a five-hour railway trip north to Parry Sound and then east on the Ottawa line into wooded country.

Dr. Richardson was a busy, hard-working country doctor who proved to be a born teacher. On the evening of my arrival he announced:

"I am sending you by horse and cutter to attend a confinement."

"But, doctor, I have never attended a confinement alone."

"You can do better than anyone else," he said. I must have looked skeptical for he added, "There is no one else there."

Though this may appear to be an addle-brained remark, it proved to be a very supporting thought then and later during many lonely assignments. I remember most particularly, as clearly as though it were yesterday, an occasion some seven years later. Mrs. K. had a sudden miscarriage at the fifth month of pregnancy. When I reached her home at 3 a.m. after a drive of six miles on a cold winter night, she was unconscious at intervals from hemorrhaging. Her husband sidled up to me saying, "Do the best you can, Doctor, we need her here." He didn't need to tell me this. The children were up and I could count—there were five. Though I was prepared for this emergency, I went outside to walk the road and to think. My concern for the patient was compounded by a peculiar feeling of resentment. It was one of the few times I felt sorry for myself. The house was on a hilltop and I could look about the countryside without a light visible for ten miles. It was eerie. There I was sweating out a problem in loneliness and anxiety when all about me people were enjoying sleep. Suddenly Dr. Richardson's dictum came to me: "No one can do better as there is no one else here." I returned with a lighter heart to my patient, to start intravenous fluids and put in a vaginal packing with a lighted speculum and long-handled forceps. The task was finished in about an hour and a half, when the bleeding stopped and the patient brightened to ask for a drink.

Dr. Richardson taught me, among other things, that there is more to doctoring than medical skill. One afternoon he accosted me: "I brought you up here to make my patients feel better. Smile! Look as though you are interested and pleased—cheerfulness is as important as pill and potion."

Another time he directed me to go six miles into the country where a horse had torn its chest open on a stake. My instructions were to do a neat careful repair with large needle and sutures and tell the owners to keep the animal out of doors the rest of the winter. I could see that Dr. Richardson viewed this as a serious mission and no time to make a facetious remark about my not being a horse doctor. The animal was one of a team of fine Clydesdales owned by a middle-aged Finnish couple who were carving out a farm in the woods. On a return visit four days later I found them very grateful and was paid five dollars for my services.

At medical school there were a number of good clinical teachers. Some, of course, were better than others, with probably about ten of them making Toronto Medical School an excellent center of instruction. These were teachers for whom we all had the deepest respect. Other lecturers, in considerable number, were satisfied just to fill our minds with facts we could have gotten from books. They appeared to be little interested in us as individuals and their attitude was: Listen to what I have to tell you and be prepared to give it back without argument at examination time. Quite a few in bedside teaching of groups limited their interest largely to the bright students or their favorites. It wasn't hard for some of us to hang back and do nothing but listen.

Dr. C. L. Starr, sitting casually on the edge of a table, could lecture so clearly on surgical problems that it seemed a waste of energy to take notes. Dr. Roscoe Graham was another master surgical teacher. In a Saturday morning class he would discuss the recorded history of some problem patient unknown to him, telling us what he thought the diagnosis would be and why. Then he would call in the surgeon on the case to tell us what was found at the operation, or the pathologist to tell us of the autopsy findings. Dr. Graham was the only teacher who exposed us to his diagnostic reasoning in this way.

Dr. J. A. Oille was a superb medical instructor. It was a delight to be in his bedside group where the slowest and brightest were all the same to him. If a student was answering his questions correctly he would persist with further questions, no matter how long it took, until the student was stuck; then he would leave him with the advice that he go home and come back next session with fresh ideas. We could never guess what he thought of our ability, but learned in time that he leaned backwards to be fair in examinations. One of my classmates in his final bedside test couldn't hear the heart murmur Dr. Oille said was present, nor would he outline the heart size on the chest wall when asked because he said he couldn't do it and if he tried, it would be his downfall. Dr. Oille quietly asked him to go home. He passed the boy, an act of sound judgment because this student went on to become a professor of the medical school.

Oral examinations for the most part were agonizing experiences for me. Possibly I had become a little proud and self-satisfied with my ability as an undergradute to pass written examinations readily where dependence upon memory was the chief factor. Oral examinations and quizzes at medical school were quite different, and adjusting to them was painfully difficult.

Dr. Alan Brown, Physician-in-Chief of the Sick Children's Hospital, Toronto, was an able instructor—a small man and a martinet. He addressed us in an amphitheatre seating about a hundred in steeply graduated rows. I was always disturbed when questioned by him in public as he called for such quick precise answers. Observing that he directed his queries mostly to those in the lower and top seats, I found it much safer to sit in the mid-section.

One famous teacher-surgeon terrified me. I couldn't think in his presence. He knocked any capacity for logical thinking clean out of me, and fate decreed that he was one of my final examiners. My comments on the swollen knee of a patient which he asked me to study must have been less than adequate as I overheard him say to a colleague behind a nearby screen, "That Johnston boy doesn't know very much, but he is going to the north country so I think I'll pass him." He was guessing that I might win by avoiding the smart city boys. This was insulting but, nevertheless, on my performance before him, I couldn't quarrel with his assessment.

There were other very able clinicians: Dr. Trevor Owen, physician, and Dr. Farrar, psychiatrist—real men and teachers they were, but I had little personal contact with them.

By graduation day I had no offers of an internship appointment, nor did I search for any. I should have done so because there is no substitute for a year's training in hospital. This was in 1923. Several years later it became mandatory to take one or two years in hospital training after finishing medical school. As preparation for practice I chose instead, as some others did, the route of spending time with one or more senior general practitioners.

First, I assisted a young doctor in Sharbot Lake, north of Kingston, Ontario. I expected to work with him out of his office, but he established me in a small nearby hamlet called Mountain Grove—a disappointment to me for I wanted to watch him at work. He was a resourceful physician and an accurate diagnostician. I helped him one morning open a young man's elbow joint and remove a loose piece of bone, with an excellent outcome. But I couldn't understand him. He looked after his patients carefully and efficiently for periods of about four weeks, when he would get a sudden urge to go to Montreal or New York—so sudden that I was called in to follow up his patients without any instructions. He was a single man who, I suspected, had an unwholesome fondness for alcohol and women. After two such absences with little warning, I quit although he offered to double my salary. Ten years later a brief newspaper item stated that this gifted but unhappy man had committed suicide by turning on a gas burner. What a pity! He had outstanding ability as a family doctor.

Next, I sought work with a busy general practitioner with teaching ability in a small city and was satisfied to stay with him a year at a salary of $100 a month plus board, with one and a half days off every six weeks. Dr. W. A. Lewis of Barrie was a competent general-practitioner surgeon. His office business methods, which required written reports of all patients, were excellent. This provided my best year of instruction and for the first time I became really enthusiastic about the practice of medicine. Furthermore, he knew how to handle me! Once when I complained of not enough responsibility he took off promptly for an afternoon of golf, leaving me to deal with a waiting room full of people. I was very relieved when the day was over, and henceforth I was ready to accept whatever rôle he assigned.

On leaving Dr. Lewis, I decided to start my own practice. But where was my big question. There was a widespread conviction among my classmates that it was injudicious to establish practice in one's home community. To this day I don't know the reasons behind this thinking. I had an attractive offer of a house with an office on Danforth Avenue in a rapidly growing section of Toronto. My prospective wife, who lived nearby on Broadview Avenue, added her words of approval to this suggestion. However, I was attracted to Lucknow as I thought I understood the ways of country folk better than city folk. Today I find this reasoning ridiculous because people are much the same anywhere in this country. Having made my decision, I resolved secretly to stay in Lucknow ten years and then move to a city, but when that time came, having encountered none of the disadvantages said to attend practice in one's home town, I concluded I wouldn't be happier anywhere else—so I stayed on.

At a cost of $4,000, with a down payment of $1,000, I bought a frame house with offices therein from a widow whose doctor-husband had died two years earlier. Father backed my loan from the local bank. Now I was ready to urge marriage to the plump attractive Toronto girl of Pennsylvania Dutch ancestry whom I had been in love with since my student days in Arts College where she was studying the classics. Perhaps I exaggerated my eagerness a little by asserting that it was now or never, but I had asked the advice of an old business friend on the subject of marriage. His answer was decisive. Banging his fist on the desk, he declared: "Young man, the time to get married is when you feel like it." I haven't heard since of a better reason.

. . . The People of Lucknow District

General medical practice is environmental medicine. To discuss it in a meaningful way calls for consideration of such things as the character of a people and their socio-economic levels—their employment, housing, incomes.

The people of the Lucknow district were the product of an interesting history. In 1615 Samuel de Champlain, with a "great War Party" of Indians, was the first white man to see the eastern shores of Lake Huron which are today's western boundaries of the Ontario counties of Huron and Bruce. He sailed up Lake Huron, which he called La Mer Douce (Freshwater Sea). Twelve years later the Jesuit Fathers from France were ministering to the 25,000 Huron Indians living along Lake Huron and eastward. The Indians developed a bitter hatred for them, not because of their teachings, but because of the measles, whooping cough and scarlet fever epidemics which accompanied their ministrations and decimated the native population.

Nothing happened during the next two hundred and twenty-five years to change the counties of Huron and Bruce from a wilderness. Then a turning point came in the 1840's. The population of Ontario (Upper Canada) nearly doubled in the decade after 1842 when it shot up from 486,000 to 950,000. This increase was due almost entirely to immigration and resulted in a demand for so much land for settlement that the supply was getting short.

At that time the 110-mile-long county of Bruce was made up of two parts. The northern peninsula area in 1836 had become an Indian reservation by the Treaty of Manitowaning. The southern part was Crown land, which with that of much of the adjoining county of Huron was known as The Queen's Bush. These Crown lands were the last unsurveyed wild lands of southern Ontario and were not opened for settlement until 1847, little more than a century ago and long after most of the rest of southern Ontario was settled. In that year surveyors marked out the roads and farms, and settlements sprang up at once. Lucknow-to-be on the Huron-Bruce boundary was right in the middle of The Queen's Bush.

Immigrants flooded into these counties from Scotland, England, Ireland and a few from Germany, setting up their semi-colonial communities. Bruce County at that time received one of the highest concentrations of Scots in the whole of Canada, mostly from the Isle of Skye, Argyll, and Sutherlandshire, where they had been evicted by their Land Clearances Act. These ordinances were designed to rid the lands of crofters to make way for sheep runs and—on the Isle of Skye—deer ranges. Those men, women and children who came to Lucknow settled mostly in the village or north and west of it, in communities that took such names as Lochalsh, Hollyrood and Kinlough.

When I arrived in Lucknow district in 1924 three-quarters of its area population were Scots. Just north of the village was a small four-square mile of hilly country know locally as The Alps, which after the trees were cleared proved to be too stony and gravelly for any crops. A Peter McKinnon was asked why his parents chose these rough hills to starve on. His answer was that after being driven from the Isle of Skye they were so pleased to be able to own any property whatever they were delighted to purchase these hills for $1.50 to $2.00 an acre.

The pioneer experiences of the Lewisites are probaly typical of the early settlements. These people, to the number of 109 families, were evicted from Lewis, the northern island of the Outer Hebrides, by a landlord so anxious to get rid of them that he paid their ship passage to the New World. They sailed in two vessels from Stornaway in 1857, arriving in Quebec City sixty-seven days later, and settled about fifteen miles northwest of Lucknow. Probably because they were extremely poor and because they were sailors and fishermen with a very rudimentary knowledge of life in this new land, their neighbors looked down on them. They suffered terribly while riding out the three-day blizzards, while learning how to lay corduroy roads through the swamps and clear the forest for planting grain. They started without horses or oxen, their only tools the axe, shovel, scythe, flail and mattock. It was a dangerous life. Many were injured and killed by falling trees and in the performance of other unaccustomed tasks, but the strong survived and the weak died off, producing hardy Canadians. After a mere fifty years there were lush gardens and meadows, fine houses, barns, roads, schools and churches to show for their labor and persistence.

There were a few settlers from other parts of Scotland. A Mr. McQuillin was insulted whenever I greeted him as a Scot. "I am not a Scotsman," he would say. "I was born in Fifeshire where I could see Edinburgh Castle on a clear day. I am a Fifer. I want you to know there was once a Kingdom of Fife." A Mrs. MacKenzie from Glasgow was wont to tell how the mothers of Glasgow in the 1850's considered they were doing well to raise half of their babies to adulthood and she marvelled at how many more would live in this land.

The Irish came by the thousands to Canada as a result of the terrible potato famines of 1846-48. During these years one and a half million Irish either died or emigrated. Another four million emigrated between the time of the famine and 1905. Many came to The Queen's Bush to settle mostly south and southwest of Lucknow in communities with such names as Dungannon, Belfast, and Donnybrook. Some of these settlers were of the Catholic faith, while others were Protestants with their flourishing temperance societies.

During the same decades there were many immigrants from

England. Their largest concentration in Huron and Bruce counties was the town of Exeter, founded by two boatloads from Devonshire. They were all Methodists, of two different brands. Some drifted north to the Lucknow area and, along with other English arrivals, started communities such as St. Helens and Whitechurch. I do not know why so many Devonshire folk came at one time. One man said his father left home because he was getting a reputation as a poacher.

Pioneers from other lands included a settlement of Alsace-Lorrainers who had a brewery at Formosa, about fifteen miles northeast of the village. North of that again were settlers from Germany in the town of Walkerton.

This mosaic of many semi-colonial communities achieved in time a quite harmonious whole. In the process the Scot, because he was greatly in the majority, was able to surround himself with much of a national character—his language, history, poetry, songs, pastimes, sports and national costume. The popular Scottish festival of January 25th, the birthday of their greatest figure, Robert Burns, was faithfully observed every year and a dance that was always part of the celebration in Lucknow brought oldsters of seventy out to kick up their heels in the *schottische*. These people had to have their own Caledonian Society, which was organized in 1875 to extend help to the needy, and became noted for the concerts, banquets, balls, and sports gatherings that attracted thousands to a grand outing on the second Wednesday in September for many years.

The site of what came to be the village of Lucknow was at the confluence of two small rivers, an area avoided by the early settlers because it was marshy and the river banks had many springs. Encircling it, however, were many pioneer settlements, and when in 1856 Eli Stauffer, a German from Waterloo county, erected a rather crude sawmill, this was the village's first building. Stauffer had been enticed by the offer of two hundred acres of free land. Two years later, lots were offered for sale in the village at a celebration marked by a salute of twenty-one guns, which were really gun-powder charges exploded in auger holes in some stately elm trees. So Lucknow came into being. Ten years later it had a population of 430 and water power was driving a sawmill, grist-mill, flour mill, and wool-carding mill. Many of its inhabitants were from the shires of Argyll and Sutherland of the Scottish Gaeldom, whose Highland troops had won fame by withstanding a Russian charge in the battle of Balaclava during the Crimean War and by crushing the Sepoy Rebellion of 1858 at Lucknow, India. The people of Bruce County had many ties of blood and friendship with the Highlanders who lifted the siege of Lucknow, India, so when the Ontario village was incorporated in 1873 it was natural to give it the name Lucknow. They went further and named all the streets after generals of the British Army serving in the Indian Mutiny: Campbell, Havelock, Rose, Canning, Ludgard are some of them. Today the roadside signs informing the traveller that he is entering Lucknow have a drawing of a horseshoe and the words "You are in Lucknow—drive Canny"; and on the reverse side "Always Welcome to our Sepoy Town."

When I started practice in Lucknow in the 1920's the county of Bruce, which had reached a peak population of 68,000 in 1891, had suffered an exodus and was down by more than one-third to 41,700. What happened? The early settlers had transmitted their pioneering blood to their children, who refused to stay put and had gone west by the thousands to help open up Western Canada. Lucknow shared in this movement; its population shrank from 1300 in 1891 to 920 in 1924.

We are concerned today with the clash of our youth with society—with the spirit of dissent that makes for misunderstanding between generations. Was this exodus to Western Canada of an earlier time a form of dissent by that generation? Is it all part of the same recurring pattern? Perhaps this dissenting sub-society of youth is sometimes the cutting edge which plows the first furrow and fells the first tree in an expanding civilization. At any rate, the youth of Bruce County of the 1890's could and did relieve their feelings of dissatisfaction by opening up new lands.

Much has been written about the characteristics of the Scots. One trait that interested me in particular was their bent for nicknames. So many were known more surely by their nicknames than by their given names that it was easier to file medical records under the former. There was a John A., a Donald A., a John and Jack in the same MacDonald family. There was Ground Hog Alex MacKenzie, who wouldn't go to school as a youngster during the winter months but resumed attendance about February 2nd when the ground hog showed itself to view the weather. There was British Lion Jack MacKenzie,* Curly Bill MacKenzie, Greasy Alex MacKenzie and Wolfie Jack MacKenzie who gave his nickname to a whole family of brothers: Wolfie Gilbert, Wolfie Neil, and Wolfie Sam. I could go on and on. There were countless others similarly characterized.

A deep respect for learning was another characteristic of the Lucknow Scots. Though they didn't talk much about it, they showed it in a number of ways. One family of four boys, with only a few years between the eldest and youngest, lost their mother when they were children and the father died when they were in their teens. They were left with little money and a small farm of a hundred acres. In a quiet discussion among themselves they decided one would train to be a carpenter, another a clergyman, another a doctor, and one would remain at home on the farm. By pooling their resources they carried out this program. The two professionals did quite well, but late in life they confided that they had made one serious mistake—that the boy left on the farm was the brainiest of the lot. Although he was a moderately successful farmer and never complained about his calling, he was not very interested in farming, preferring scholastic pursuits. Yet he stayed and was faithful to his obligations.

The Scots showed their respect for training and education in another way. When they called in a carpenter to build a staircase, they wouldn't tell him how to build it; that was his business. If they didn't like his work, they just wouldn't have him back. Nor did they ever question my handling of an illness, and

* Incidentally, this Jack MacKenzie acquired his cognomen as a result of escorting around the countryside for two years a stallion named "British Lion."

often I wouldn't know whether my services were satisfactory until another illness occurred. Even when a patient was progressing poorly they rarely made suggestions. This was in contrast to the Irish and English (and I am English-Irish) who were forever looking over my shoulder and often couldn't forego the temptation to comment and advise. Like a farmer of Irish extraction whose son was suffering from the mild eye infection known as pink eye. When it was a little slow in clearing up, the father in all sincerity made the outlandish proposal that he put some of his own urine in the eye to hurry the healing.

The Scots loved honesty. An oldster of eighty drove to the office fifteen miles one cold winter's day to greet me belligerently: "You promised two days ago to send me some medicine. I haven't received it."

"That is true," I said. "I forgot about it until this morning when I mailed it. I apologize."

"I came in to see you. I thought you would lie to me. You didn't. That is important. Please, may I shake your hand."

The Lucknow citizenry took their community obligations, religion and politics seriously. Most of the Scots were Liberals while many of the English and Irish were Conservatives, and each stayed that way.

In a community devoted largely to farming, one of the most hazardous of occupations, the people of Lucknow entered enthusiastically into their fall fairs, public auctions, barn raisings, church festivals, family reunions and even their funerals. They filled the churches to file past the dead in open coffins. Though a memorial service does soften the harshness of death, I used to regard this as a sort of pagan ritual. I am now not so sure. Viewing in this manner the body of a departed neighbor was in the nature of a last respectful meeting. At times the dead are as close to us as the living, or so my neighbors seemed to believe. I think this is one of the things they were trying to say in their memorial services. If you think this ridiculous, may I remind you that a house with a corpse in it was never empty to our ancestors.

The art and science of saving money has always been a characteristic of the Scots. Among many memorable area characters the most unforgettable one is Greasy Alex MacKenzie or Dirty Alex Mackenzie. Both the names by which he was known sum up his personal habit of living. As well as being a miser, he was unwashed. His skin had a dark brownish hue with a dull sheen and the swarthy complexion of his face and neck was characteristic of those who rarely wash.

His means of saving money were many and varied. For years his contribution to the Sunday service was a copper on the plate. In late mid-life he developed a small cancer on the upper tip of one ear lobe. This lesion is easy to cure by excision, as it does not spread until after many months of growth. But Alex was pretty worried about it and his physician sent him to the Mayo Clinic in Rochester, Minnesota. His doctor told me that Alex had a new suit of clothes for this visit, but took along a suit of dirty work clothes. When ready to leave he put on the dirty worn outfit to enquire about his account. They politely informed him they did not know what his bill was and that they would mail it in a few days. Later he received an account for $500; he hadn't deceived the clinic.

At the age of 76 he was ill with pneumonia under the care of his niece, a trained and competent nurse, in her farmhouse. After several days she reported that, "Alex is eating poorly and I have an idea that he may be worrying about paying extra for his food. Could you tell him that his meals are included in my fee for looking after him?" I tried out her suggestion.

"Alex, I am worried about your not eating. You are in the fortunate position of paying the same for your care whether you eat or not." It worked. He ate more with the next meal and with good food and the aid of penicillin he made an excellent recovery.

He was an interesting but not a very likeable patient. The first occasion he consulted me was about a sore on his shin. In my surgery I found my first task was to wash his leg to find the ulcer. It was a new experience to see how dirty a leg could be and how high it could smell. When he went out, I aired the office by opening both windows and doors. I put an elastoplast dressing around his leg.

"Doctor, how much do I owe you?"

"Two dollars, Alex."

"Will you take what I have in my wallet sight unseen? It might be more than that or it might be less; it's all the money I have with me."

"I don't think so, Alex. You will be in town again in a few days." He emptied out his small dirty black purse on my table and its grimy coins added up to $1.21. He put them back and after chatting a few minutes got up to go.

"Doctor, how much do I owe you?"

"Two dollars, Alex."

He put his hand in another pocket and drew out a fistful of bills from which he peeled off a two-dollar bill. He was getting absent-minded and had forgotten his earlier discussion of the fee.

One summer evening I gave him a lift in my car as he was walking to his home one mile from the village. He was carrying a loaf of bread and a chunk of cheese and told me he had just broken a bottle of milk by dropping it on the paved road. He wouldn't let me drive him back for another bottle. "This accident will be a lesson to me to be more careful."

He was a small man of about five feet six in height, and 150 pounds weight, which belied his toughness and great strength. He wore large coarse shoes and dressed in plain heavy work clothes with the sleeves and neck of the coat scuffed and dirty. On cold winter days he might sometimes wear an overcoat, but more often not, appearing to be inadequately clad. Rainy weather or snow storms would not keep him indoors if there was anything of advantage to do outdoors. He was always on the move, appearing to be intent on going some place in a hurry. It was difficult to engage him in a few minutes of casual street conversation.

"Dirty Alex" came from a large family. His father died when he was a child. He never married. His brothers, sisters, half-brothers and half-sisters all left home and he remained with his mother to carry on the home farm. She faithfully looked after the house for him. She was a sad-looking, dowdy woman and no wonder. She was treated as a chattel and never had any money to spend. But managing the farm soon wasn't enough for Alex, and he started helping the neighbors on a daily payment basis. He liked physical labor and was known as a fast, capable and faithful workman, always giving more of his energies than was called for. The days weren't long enough for him. He would continue cutting his grain until dark and the following morning the neighbors would note that it was now all neatly stooked and sometimes even a part of it in the barn. On the death of his mother, in his early mid-life, he sold the farm and bought a small cottage near the village where he became his own housekeeper. Now he depended entirely on working for others as an unskilled workman and thought nothing of walking many miles morning and evening for a day's work. He never owned a car.

With all his avarice, he was known as an honest man. I never heard that he ever demanded what was not his. When a mortgagor failed to make a payment on the due date, Alex might appear early at his door the next morning to enquire what was the matter. But in looking for payments from those owing him money, he was not considered to be hard or harshly exacting.

In 1939 one of Dirty Alex's few confidants informed me that he wished to make a Will. He had the details typed out and he wanted me to go out and see Alex and when I found him of sound mind or *compos mentis*, as the legal term states, then we would both visit him for his signature.

We both knew this provision of Will-making was overdue, as he was getting senile. Three years earlier I had brought him to his cottage late at night from a railway station 20 miles distant. On returning from a brother's funeral in Detroit, he had got off at the wrong station and didn't know were he was. Also, there were innumerable reports going back several years of people finding Alex wandering hopelessly lost and confused miles from his home.

Certifying to his testamentary capacity posed a real problem. Was he sane enough to make a Will which would stand up in a court of law? The provisions of the Will made it quite likely that some of the relatives would contest it.

Somewhere I had learned that you don't need to know very much to make a Will. You just have to be able to answer three questions:

i) What are your possessions?
ii) Who are your close relatives?
iii) What do you wish to leave each of them?

I made three early morning visits to his cottage to get better acquainted and particularly to judge his sanity. I concluded that his forgetfulness with some degree of mental confusion was not constant. They were of the intermittent type. It was plain to me that Dirty Alex could be clear-witted when rested, and very muddled when weary and exhausted, especially late in the day.

Medical literature showed that some authorities believed that forgetfulness of the intermittent type is characteristic of senile brain changes due to hardened arteries. On my third morning visit I found his mind quite clear. I brought his friend out at once and in his presence read the Will to Alex clause by clause. It was unique.

Only two or three of his brothers, sisters, half brothers and half sisters remained alive and he said none of them were in need. He left each of them one dollar. In explanation he said, "They have had no use for me when I was alive and I'll have no use for them when I'm dead." He was under the mistaken impression that he had to leave these relatives something and that the minimum possible was one dollar. It was a shrewd action as it proved to any reader that the named beneficiaries had not been forgotten. He made some substantial bequests to a number of nieces and nephews and to two local churches. The residue of his estate was left to establish a fund from which Lucknow high school boys could obtain interest-free loans for further studies.

Like most of his race, Alex had a deep respect for education. He gave the impression that he regretted having had very little schooling of any kind. Feeling inferior in this respect may have driven him to prove his worth in some field—that of piling up money. Also, his money bundle gave him some status in the community. It was obvious that he had no regrets about his lifelong miserly living. He said, "I hope they have as much fun spending it as I had making it." Also, keeping some of his money intact and at the same time out of the hands of government may have appealed to his mercenary instincts.

When he made his Will, the estate had shrunk from a high of $125,000 to $100,000, due to the operations of the Farmer's Credit Arrangements Act. This Act during the depression of the early 1930's—the so-called dirty 30's—drastically scaled down the mortgages of many farmers, including a few held by Alex. Nevertheless, there was $60,000 left for the High School Students' Loan Fund.

Immediately after his death in April 1943 some of the surviving relatives set out to break the Will on the grounds of mental incompetence. They had no difficulty mustering dozens of witnesses to prove the confusion and forgetfulness of his later years. The hearing was before a trial judge without a jury in the Surrogate Court of the County of Bruce.

The Judge found that Alex lacked testamentary capacity. It was then taken to the Ontario Court of Appeal which reversed the Judge's decision. Finally, it was reviewed by the Chief Justices of the Supreme Court of Canada who upheld the Will.

By this time the residue of the estate to the Lucknow High School Fund had decreased further to $39,000. Since its establishment, this Fund has been drawn upon by needy students to the maximum extent. I am told it is the only high school in Canada with such a local fund. In 1969 the terms of assistance from the Will were changed by the Supreme Court from granting interest-free loans to that of bursaries for bright students.

Incidentally I have been told that the Judges were impressed by my action of visiting Alex three times before deciding that his mind was clear enough to discuss and understand his Will, and that this case has become a precedent in this branch of the law.

Misers never have been described as admirable people. Samuel Johnson expressed some of this feeling when he said, "It is easy to make money if you lower your mind to it." This would place "Dirty Alex," an expert in money-grubbing and miserliness, pretty low in the scale of humans. But why moralize at all about an individual with such marked plus and minus elements? All his actions were not selfish and reprehensible. Rest his soul.

These were some of the characteristics of the vigorous and competent people of Lucknow district among whom I cast my lot. They had, of course, the common failings. There was always the controversial matter of drinking. In the twenties, the overuser of alcohol was the town drunk; we never called him an alcoholic, and we never considered him ill. He was an unfortunate who had fallen off the water wagon and nothing more. If he was combative, or simply obnoxious, the local police saw to it that he slept it off in the cold lockup of the town hall.

What citizens thought individually of the use and abuse of alcohol depended partly on their ethnic background. On one occasion I twitted a Scottish farmer: "Why does every Scot household in this area have a supply of whiskey?"

"Well, Doctor," was his reply, "Prohibition is only for those not strong enough to handle alcohol."

One of our leading merchants was a successful and highly respected owner-manager of a grocery and feed store. Every Saturday evening he invited his intimate friends to his office for a drink—and he was liberal with it. There was nothing boisterous about the gathering, just a quiet generous sharing of the contents of a bottle. This same man was one of the local preachers in the Free Church of Scotland that served the Lucknow area in the absence of professional clergy, and he was obliged to conduct the Sunday morning service at 11 a.m. He rarely missed and I never heard a breath of criticism from the parishioners about his fondness for liquor, although it was openly admitted that one could tell on Sunday how much he had imbibed the previous evening by the length of his prayers—the more alcohol, the longer the prayers.

An elderly retired citizen of Scots parentage reported this experience which occurred when he was a lad of 19 and about to leave the village on his first away-from-home employment as a bank clerk. A local clergyman of the Free Church of Scotland learned of his early employment and left word that he wished to see him. The young man went to his home and met the clergyman in a room he called his office. On his desk was a bottle of whiskey from which he poured a glass to offer his young visitor with these words, "I want to advise you that this may be the most helpful or the most dangerous stuff in the world. It can lift you out of a serious depression or it can ruin you completely if its usage is uncontrolled." He hadn't a word of advice about abstinence—just suggested learning how to use it wisely.

My elderly retired friend comments that he thinks his reverend advisor was a bit of a hypocrite as he later heard him preach strongly against any use of alcoholic beverages.

In contrast, there was Tom Cain, an Irishman known as "Old Goddamnit," the owner and manager of the Cain House, the village hotel. "Whiskey should never be drunk—it should only be sold," was one of his sayings. He was never known to drink a drop. Another of his homilies was, "I always know when cold weather is here—the flies go out and the bums come in."

Huron County on one side of the village with its citizenry of English and Irish extraction, unlike Bruce County on the other side, was one of the temperance strongholds of Canada. Early in this century many Ontario counties adopted the Canada Temperance Act (CTA) of 1878, which was regarded as quite a successful piece of legislation with its ban on all sales of alcoholic beverages. One after another, the various Ontario counties rescinded the Act when the Ontario government started its liquor control legislation after the Prohibition period of 1916-1926. One of the last to do so was Huron County in 1959. In contrast, Bruce County—with its high percentage of citizenry of Scots ancestry—voted for the CTA in 1885 but after a trial of only four years gave it up for good.

A community without differences in tastes and habits would be intolerably bland. Lucknow district was anything but that. I found its people diverse and full of flavor.

II. Before the Age of Miracles: Some Instructive First Steps

Starting out in the medical world on my own in 1924, I soon found that I knew much more than I realized and much less than my patients thought I knew.

My first patient was an elderly widower whom I called on in the evening for a severe right-sided pain from a kidney stone. He was given a hypodermic of morphine. Next morning he couldn't thank me enough. My reaction was surprise at the ease with which I had brought him relief. I was thrilled that a simple hypo could do so much. Of course, he required further study in hospital to bring permanent relief but this could be done leisurely and in relative comfort.

A child named Tommy was my first dramatic cure.

The thyroid gland in our neck produces a hormone which has a profound effect on growth and development. It has been called "the draft of the fire of metabolism." In some instances it creates illness by producing excessive amounts of hormone, and in other instances by producing too little hormone, and occasionally none at all. An infant born lacking this hormone is in a disastrous situation. The blazing fire of young life is dampened and the child becomes an idiot, a hopelessly deficient creature called a cretin. This type of idiocy was first recognized about 1860 in England and was one of the first forms of mental retardation found to be preventable.

Tommy at three months was a lazy feeder, with a bulging belly button and a protruding tongue. I considered him to be a cretin and started giving him small daily doses of thyroid extract—first an eighth of a grain, then a quarter grain, and occasionally half a grain. He changed rapidly and in two years he was a very different looking boy. He was kept on small daily doses of thyroid extract and at ten years he needed none at all, or only an eighth of a grain daily which is an unusually small dosage for this type of patient. At that time he was in Grade IV in public school, getting A's and B's, and quite athletic. Tommy really excited me. I used to make excuses to visit his home in the country just to listen to what the parents had to say about their boy. It was a disappointing day for me when the family moved away. I truly missed Tommy.

One could say that I was emotionally involved with Tommy. Which raises questions often asked me: Is there danger of the family doctor becoming too emotionally involved with his patients for his own effectiveness? And if so, how did I meet it? To the first question I would say: Yes, there is such a danger, although I doubt I would call it a major hazard. I felt a very personal concern about Tommy, it is true, but it didn't affect my performance as his physician—and fortunately the outcome was happy. Emotional involvement with a patient doomed to death is different and can be so exhausting as to impair a doctor's power to be of service. It depends to some extent upon temperament.

One of my classmates, a close friend, confided that he couldn't keep from worrying unduly over seriously ill patients. At the age of forty-five he found himself unable to sleep when he had a patient who was dangerously ill. My friend at that time looked prematurely old; he died a few years later. Another classmate in Detroit, I have been told, suddenly changed from medical practice to another vocation after the unexpected deaths of three patients.

As for me—after a particularly trying illness, it was a wonderful restorative of spirit to disappear into the country for an evening of poker or bridge where only an emergency could reach me. It was better still if I could go off for a holiday.

I had not practiced many years when I decided to attend no more funerals of my patients—even of close friends. I found them so depressing that my effectiveness in bringing cheer and hope into a sickroom was compromised for a period of time. Occasionally my wife would accuse me of being cold and unfeeling, but I couldn't bear listening to the words of sympathy and solace that were an accepted part of the ritual. To be told that the death of a young man or woman from a vicious disease was the Lord's will invariably shocked me. Such a death was, to me, due to our ignorance and I could only remember the young person's bitter frustration, his feeling of being cheated that life should end so soon. I had to believe that the Lord permitted these deaths, but he didn't will them; instead, he willed that we use our brains and talents to prevent and cure illness and postpone death.

The miracle of birth I was to experience many times, under varying conditions. I remember in my novice days sitting in a hospital labor room looking at a newborn boy who wasn't breathing. He had a *meningocele*—a lump on his lower back as large as my fist. This meant he might have hopelessly paralyzed legs. The mother was a schoolteacher in her mid-thirties. It was her first pregnancy, and she was so anxious to have a baby that she would be heartbroken to see it a helpless cripple. Was it a kindness to bring the child into the world? I was in my second year of practice and had never before faced a situation like this. I watched the infant for what seemed an appreciable interval, but was probably only a minute or two, wondering what to do . Then I remarked to the nurses, "It is my business to save life." With a little effort the boy was soon breathing.

A few months later a surgeon removed the lump and fortunately found only a few of the nerves to one leg curled up in it. The boy grew into a bright lad and it was thrilling to see him tripping to school past my office with a scarcely perceptible limp. Never again did I hesitate to keep a young life going.

It was unusual that this birth had taken place in the hospital. Most births in those years were in the home. It was not until well after the mid-twenties that hospital confinements became popular and I could refuse to accept pregnant patients unless they agreed to go into hospital. Hospital rounds meant a great deal of travel, often under trying circumstances. Wingham Hospital was ten miles east, Kincardine twenty miles north, and Goderich twenty-two miles southwest, and at times I had patients in all three. Eventually I insisted on using only Wingham Hospital. Though I lost some patients by this decision, my practice became more manageable.

Some admission figures to Wingham Hospital are interesting. Mrs. Iris Morrey, administrator of the hospital, has provided the following information about admissions for the year 1920. Wingham was a town of 3,000 and its hospital served an area population of 10,000 to 12,000. The town had two capable resident general-practitioner surgeons at the time.

Year	*Surgical*	*Medical*	*Obstetrical*	*Total*
1920	140	24	17	198 (Includes 17 babies)

The Surgical Diagnoses:

Tonsils and Adnoids removal	45
Appendectomies	29
Appendectomies and Cholecystectomies	3
Cholecystectomies (gall bladder operation)	1
Abscesses drained:	13
Appendix — 5	
Axilla — 1	
Bladder — 1	
Neck — 2	
Breast — 3	
R — leg — 1	
Accidents:	11
Fractured Tibia — 3	
Fractured Femur — 1	
Injuries to Hand — 4	
Injuries to Face — 1	
Injuries to Eye — 2	
Circumcision	2
Hernia Repair	12
Hysterectomy	7
Gastro-enterology	3

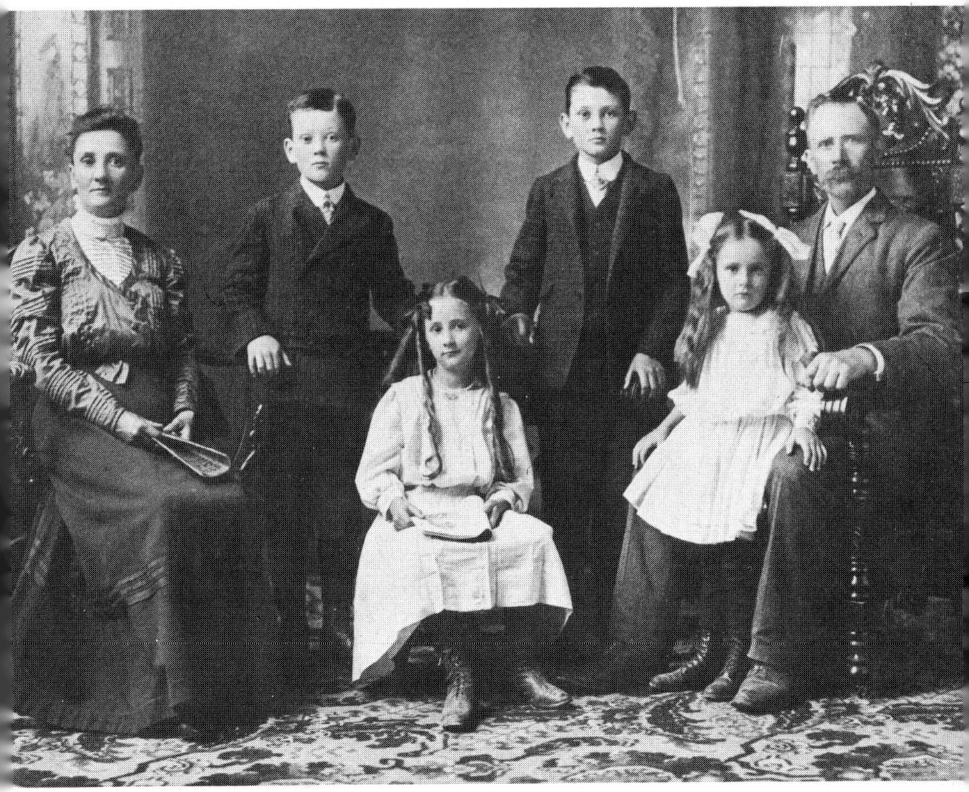

The Albert E. Johnston family in 1910.

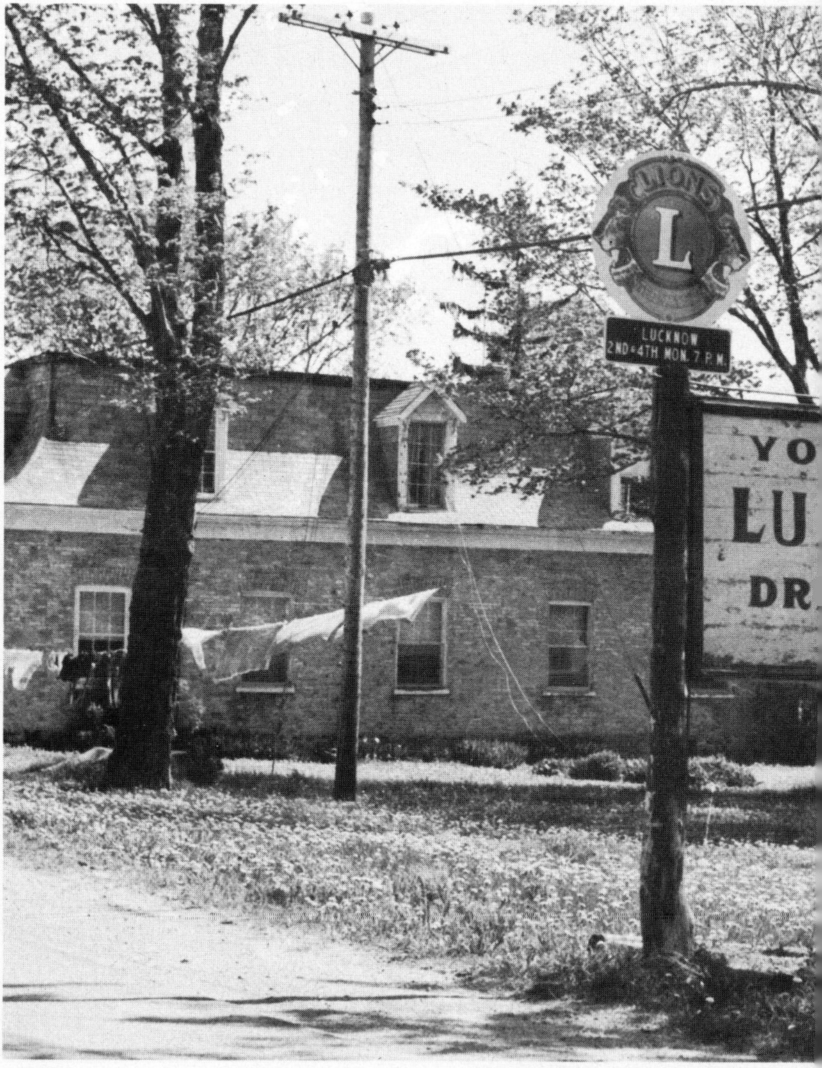

Highway sign at entrance to the village of Lucknow. It was sometimes called the Sepoy town in allusion to the Anglo-Indian word for a native soldier of the British Army at the time of the Indian mutiny (which included the relief of the city of Lucknow).

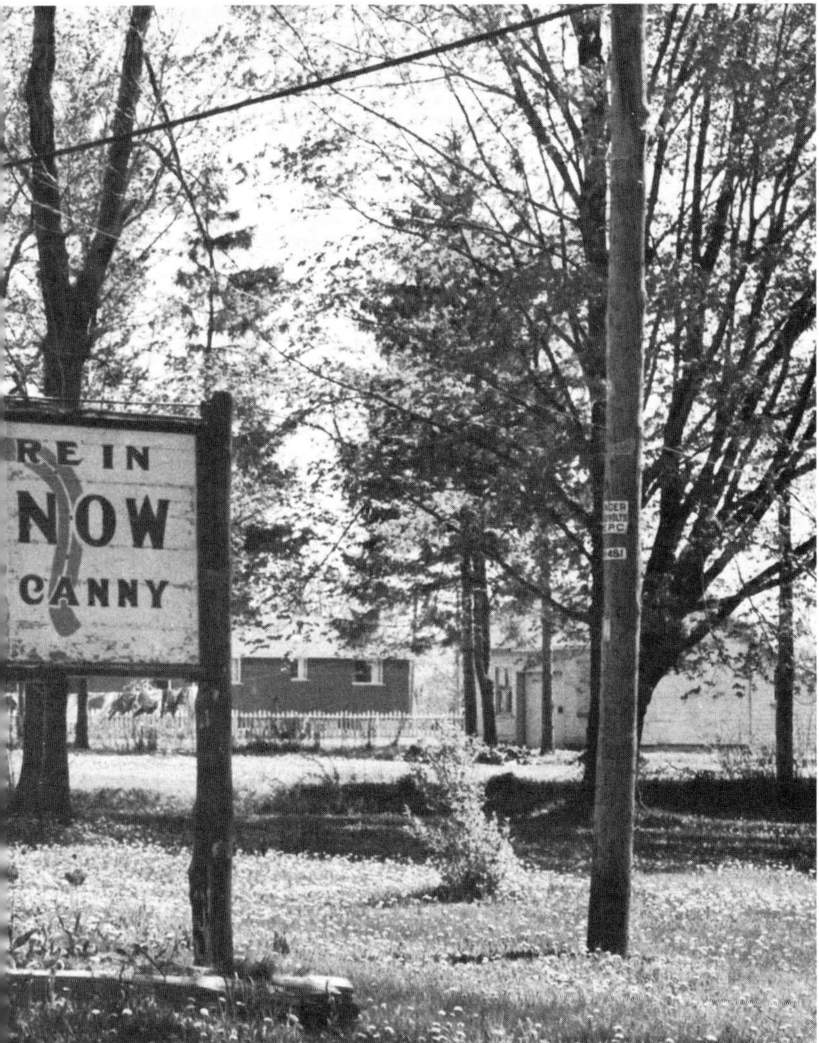
RE IN
NOW
CANNY

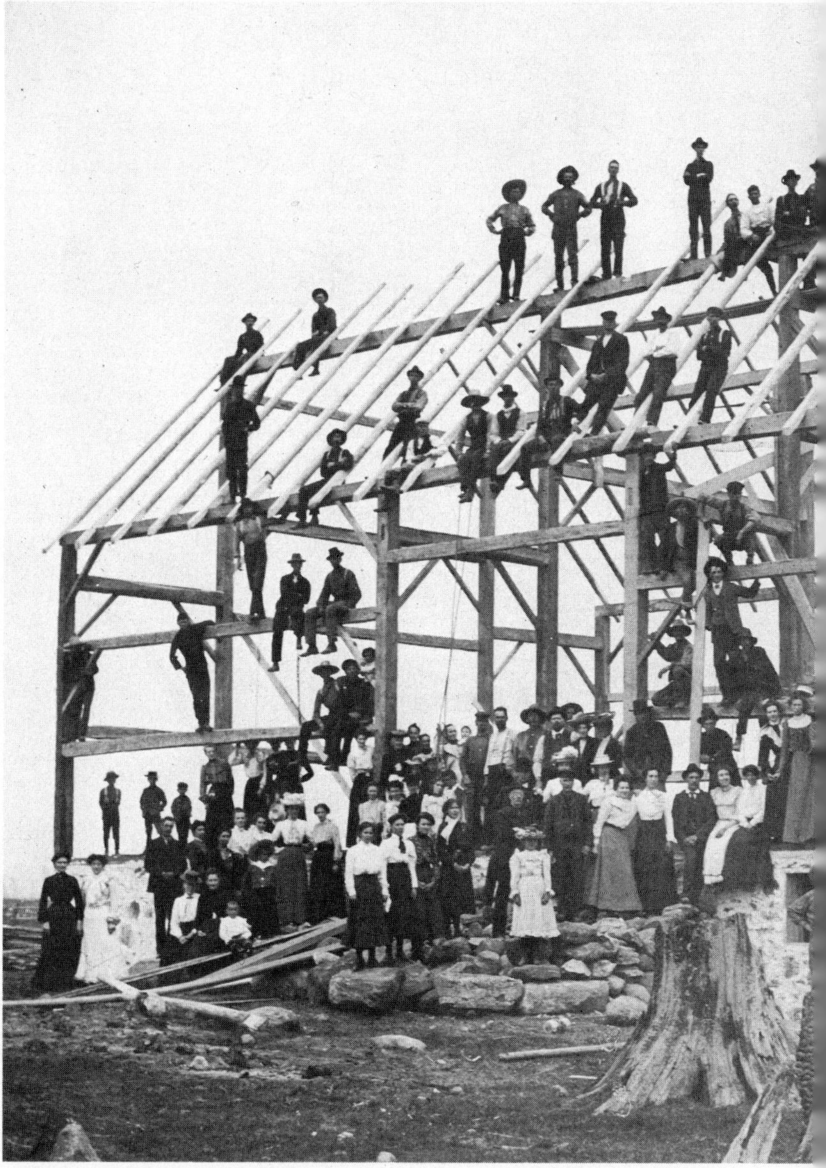

A barn raising such as the one illustrated here was Dr. Johnston's first conscious event as a child.

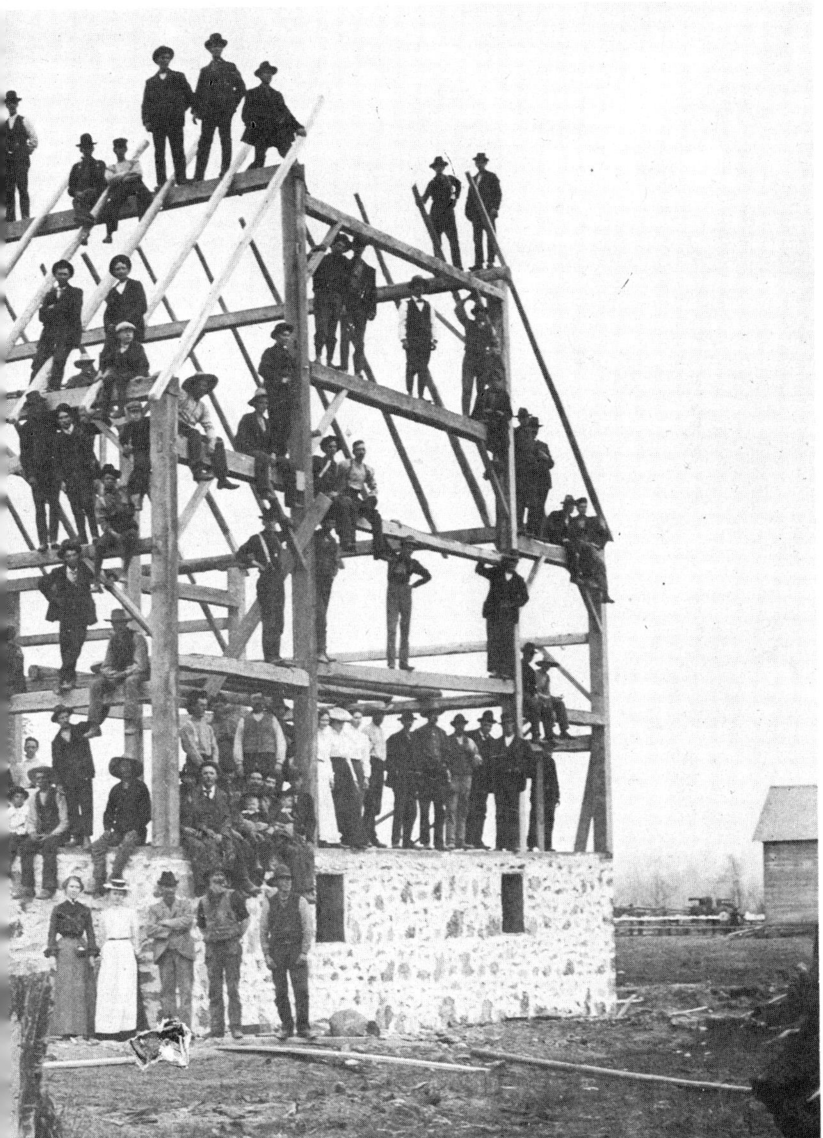

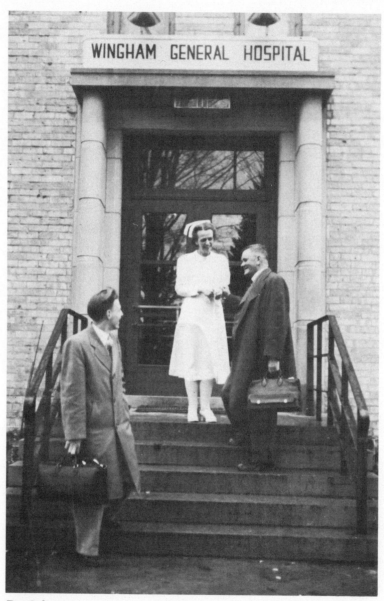

Dr. Johnston with his associate Dr. Melvin Corrin and Hospital Superintendant Mrs. Iris Morrey.

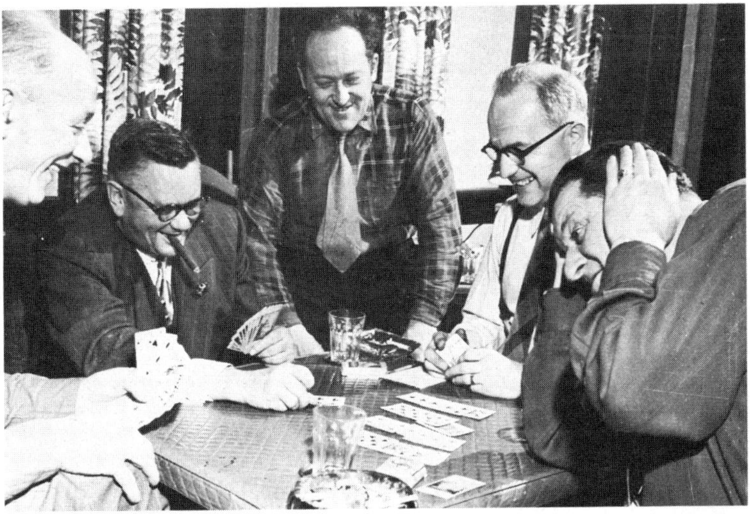

The author playing a relaxing game of bridge with friends on a night away from the office.

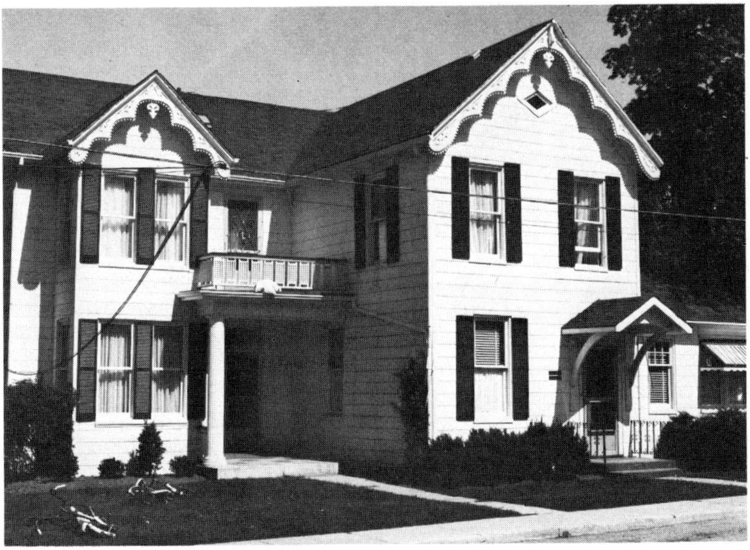

Dr. Johnston's house in Lucknow with entrance to his office at right of photograph.

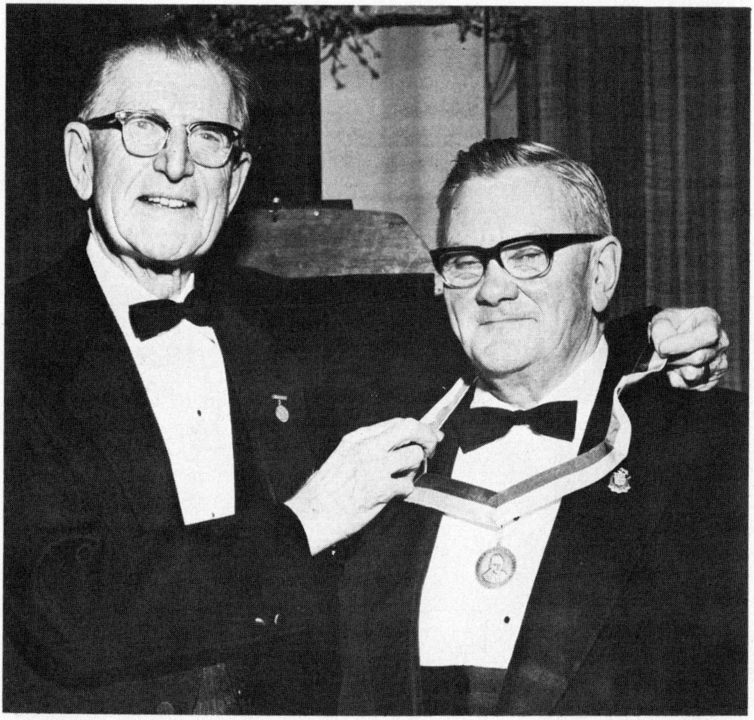

The author is shown here being presented with the William Victor Johnston Medal of Honor which was struck by the College of General Practice in 1965. Making the presentation is Charles Gass, a past president of the college.

D & C	4
Ectopic Gestation .... (misplaced pregnancy)	2
Hemorrhoid Operation	1
Nasal Septum Resection	3
Fistula-in-ano	1
Inguinal Hernia	1
Trachelorrhaphy .... (Suture of cervix)	1
Thyroidectomy	1
	38
TOTAL	140

(You will note that though there was considerable major surgery, quite a high percentage of the hospital surgery of that year would be classified today as minor in nature.)

The following figures on admissions tell a little of the story of the change that took place over three decades:

Year	*Surgical*	*Medical*	*Obstetrical*	*Total*
1920	140	24	17	181
1925	129	48	28	205
1930	113	44	42	199
1935	123	51	36	210
1940	149	96	77	322
1950	358	716	216	1,290

(You will note that in earlier years, the surgical admissions far exceeded the medical and obstetrical, while by 1950 the trend was almost reversed.)

Confinements in the home could present many problems. I recall vividly one late bitter night when a Mr. G. came into the office, so worried he could scarcely speak coherently. His wife was in labor and their doctor, an alcoholic confrère, was on a bender. Would I come? I hesitated. It was snowing and blowing so hard that the three-mile side road might be impassable. Or I might get through with the car by lucky driving and by gunning the motor with a risk of serious damage to it. It was no comfort to recall that Mr. G. had the reputation of being unpleasant to anyone asking for payment of goods or services. But I had to think of his wife. I knew her to be a bright, cheerful woman, all heart for her four children, even though she was not very logical or provident. A doctor called in a case of emergency must be helpful to a maximum degree; there is really no neutral ground for him to stand on. Here was a woman with little sunshine in her life, who probably deserved a better fate than being married to a shiftless husband.

As a final inducement, Mr. G. came to a decision and made a rare offer:

"Doctor, what will your fee be?"

"Twenty-five dollars, Mr. G."

"I will pay you as soon as it is over."

We arrived safely at his home after some tricky driving. I didn't know that such squalor and cold existed. The mother was lying on a couch in the bedroom covered only by a thin quilt and her coat. Her face and hands were dirty. One stone wall of the basement was caved in and the wind howled through this hole to whistle up through the cracks of the bedroom floor. The practical nurse with me soon had a fire roaring in the wood stove. The children had punched holes through the plaster wall above the mother's couch through which to watch proceedings. I threw a pillow against the peepholes, but when newer and larger ones soon appeared I gave up.

The baby was born without undue difficulty. In the absence of clothing, it was wrapped in rags. Mr. G. was as good as his word and promptly peeled off from a roll twenty-five one-dollar bills. On my return next day with clothing donated by my wife and friends, both baby and mother were thriving, though the house was still bitterly cold.

Experiences amid such cold and abject poverty were rare as we had few really poor people in the district. Even that, however, is regrettable in a country as rich as ours. Only one other birth in a cold and draughty bedroom comes to mind. On that occasion the nurse drew my attention to the "steam" rising from the new-born infant, as from one's breath on a sub-zero morning. The mother went out the next day to milk the cow.

Every doctor must be prepared for surprises, pleasant as well as unpleasant. Attending a pregnant woman ten miles north of the village was a pleasant and enlightening experience even if a little wearying. Arriving at her home on a Saturday evening, I stayed all night. There was no nurse with me this time, and I didn't dare leave. The baby was born Sunday afternoon at 4 p.m., weighing 6½ pounds. It was then I discovered there was another waiting in line. While I bided my time the mother turned over and went to sleep. At 10 p.m. she roused herself, was in labor again and had the second child two hours later—six pounds this time. This was my first birth of twins; it was precisely like two separate confinements. Eventually I was to attend more than my share of multiple births—nearly three score.

Speaking of twins, a rather interesting incident comes to mind. I did my own tonsillectomies because I believed I could perform them expertly. For more than twenty years I had no complications whatever from this operation, such as bleeding a few hours later.

Then one morning I removed the tonsils of twin girls about 10 years of age. After repeated attacks of sore throat I thought their tonsils hadn't returned to a completely healthy state and were still harboring streptococcus germs. General practitioners are sometimes accused of removing too many tonsils. We removed a considerable number because we found from experience it gave most of these children better health.

Everything went without incident in the removal of the tonsils of these twins and each left the operating room with a dry throat. In the late afternoon one of them had considerable oozing from one tonsil bed and back in the operating room the bleeding vessel was tied. Later that evening the twin sister was showing some difficulty in breathing. Her throat was filling up with a huge blood clot in one tonsil bed and all the surface tissue around it and up onto the palate was black from blood oozing into it. I hadn't seen anything like this before.

Under anaesthesia the blood clot was removed. That is all that was necessary. Both these girls were saved from possible disaster by prompt action, the first one might very well have died from bleeding and the other from suffocation.

We frequently read in the news where identical twins in mid and later life and living far apart become ill at the same time with similar afflictions. It seems to me that here we had a similar strange occurrence.

It is obvious that the human race is very durable, particularly its women. The mind boggles trying to assess the amazing strength of women in childbirth down through the ages in all parts of the world and under the most trying conditions: the Eskimo mother who goes out on the ice alone to have her baby, the English women during the Middle Ages and our own Canadian pioneer mothers.

The art of obstetrics has evolved slowly. The Hindus had midwives—four to a mother—and knew a lot about the stages of pregnancy. It was their custom to tie off the umbilical cord and hang it about the neck of the child. The Greeks had a kind of midwife so trained that physicians attended only difficult labors —which we are told constituted three out of every five, and this among an athletic race.

By 1920, major obstetrical advances had been made. The pioneer in antisepsis, Semmelweis, in May 1847 had introduced chlorine water in the wards of the Vienna hospitals and the deaths from childbed fever dropped within a year from 12 to 1.2 per cent. Semmelweis was driven from Vienna, but antisepsis was soon accepted all over the Western world. Then followed a long period of emphasis on non-interference as a policy in labor: Leave nature alone except when definite complications appear. I was a cautious, even timid obstetrician, both by training and by choice.

In obstetrical practice, one of the most terrifying things we had to deal with in the twenties was pre-eclamptic convulsions. Though very dangerous to both mother and child, they were largely preventable by monthly examinations involving among other things a search for albumen in the urine. But despite efforts to popularize the idea of monthly check-ups, it took years to educate women to the importance of this program.

Dr. George E. Case of Newmarket was admonishing a woman threatened with convulsions whose urine was loaded with albumen. "Why didn't you come earlier?"

Her husband spoke up: "Doctor, each of her two earlier babies came with the second fit." Here was a woman who had had convulsions with each of three pregnancies.

Some of the older general physicians had a lot of knowledge about this hazard and unique ways of dealing with it. My senior village colleague one morning received a sample of urine from one of his maternity patients. After testing it he rushed to the woman's home, packed her in steaming hot blankets and, after waiting long enough to see that she was in a good sweat, he said, "My dear, I suppose you would like to go to Teeswater Fall Fair this afternoon."

"I certainly would," she agreed.

"You may go if you will come home early."

The woman went to the fair, enjoyed herself, and the next morning was delivered of what appeared to be a normal child. I am reasonably sure of this—he is my son-in-law.

The same practitioner called me out to a farmhouse one winter's evening to assist with a young woman of eighteen in convulsions with her first pregnancy—an alarming situation. She was near full term but not in labor. When I learned what he proposed to do, I was apprehensive and even frightened. As he explained the procedure to me, I would sit at the end of the kitchen table on which the young woman lay and slowly pour drops of chloroform onto gauze over her nose while he dilated her cervix and delivered the baby. I had been taught never to attempt this procedure with such a dangerously toxic woman. It was a perilous undertaking and condemned without reservations by all my instructors and textbook authorities.

In the next three hours the doctor did what he had planned. He manually dilated the cervix by alternating right and left hands as they tired and neatly, carefully delivered a six-pound baby. The mother had no more convulsions and was up doing her housework after the usual ten-day period of rest. It was a masterful performance by any standards.

One swallow doesn't make a summer and I was never tempted to try such a risky operation myself. Nevertheless, I had to respect my confrère's resourcefulness and skill. Some experienced family doctors of those days were very talented.

The approved treatment of this toxic condition before convulsions developed was rest in bed—the most important measure—a salt-free diet, and estimation of the blood pressure once or twice a day. If the condition stabilized and the baby still seemed healthy, the mother was left alone. But if the blood pressure continued to rise we tried to induce labor with quinine and pituitrin. Should that not produce successful results, the membranes were ruptured. This was usually effective, but if not the situation was desperate and a Caesarean birth might be undertaken. Dr. E. K. Lyon of Leamington, Ontario, describes his treatment:

"In the treatment of pre-eclamptic convulsions, these patients were put to bed. They were put on a low-salt diet, chiefly liquids with plenty of milk, and an attempt was made, if they were near term, to get them into labor. This was carried out by rupturing the membranes or sometimes without even rupturing the membranes, by the insertion of a Voorhee's bag. Following this insertion they were given castor oil, then quinine, and periodically the nurse or attendant was instructed to give a little tug on the Voorhee's bag to attempt to stimulate uterine contractions.

"It was surprising how often this method of inducing labor was successful. I had a series of bags of various sizes. As I recall, there were four sizes, starting with one approximating a cervix barely dilated. As the patient expelled one bag a larger one was put in. When eclampsia became full-blown with convulsions the patient was given morphine in a hospital and put in a dark room. As early as the 1920's we were using intramuscular magnesium sulfate to control convulsions." It was known, even then, that assault of Caesarean section, when the patient was already ill, was not good treatment, although it was being done by some of the senior men accustomed to believe that immediately the uterus was emptied all the problems were solved. We know, of course, that this is not true because a certain number of these patients develop eclamptic convulsions as late as one or two days after delivery.

My most unfortunate experience of this terrible affliction was with a woman of thirty-five who had had one healthy child. She entered hospital at the sixth month in convulsions. In spite of everything we tried, it was six weeks later before the baby was born, fortunately alive and well. But the mother's health was permanently damaged. Her brain had been so injured from the long session with high blood pressure that she was like an old person following several "strokes."

Childbirth is one of the most common conditions the family doctor is called upon to treat, and one of the most fascinating—offering the most tangible rewards. In the twenties we liked to use chloroform as an anaesthetic, though we later changed to ether. We recognized that with its use there was a narrow margin between safety and danger—a risk of death about 1 in 1000. We gave it without a mask, just drop by drop on a small square of gauze over the nose—that is, lots of air with it. Morphine was also a marvellous drug on occasion. One G.P. tells me how he sat all day in a home from eight in the morning till nine at night watching a woman with her twelfth baby. The cervix wouldn't dilate, she was too nervous and tense. As the woman raised strong objections to his leaving, he gave her a quarter grain of morphine; the cervix flew open and the baby was born in ten minutes.

In the 1920's Canadian doctors had not begun to experiment with working together in partnerships or groups. I learned early in my practice that nurses were the doctors' best friends—both practical and registered nurses, including midwives. For the first two or three years my wife attended the office telephone, until I engaged a nurse at ten dollars a week to handle the office routine and help with patients. The community had a reasonably adequate supply of what were called practical nurses, mostly middle-aged women without formal training but with a natural aptitude for caring for the sick. They assisted at many home confinements, and looked after patients not requiring hospitalization—and understandably they were in constant demand.

There was considerable nursing in both home and hospital for graduate nurses. My major surgery was performed by consultant surgeons usually in the hospital, but sometimes on the kitchen table in the home. One nurse, Miss Elva Johnston, was especially helpful with home surgery. All she needed was about two hours' time to wash the floor and woodwork of the kitchen, ready sterile pillows, sheets and dressings, see to facilities for the anaesthetist, make sure of good lighting and basins for the surgeon. Never did I see any ill effects from a well-planned kitchen table operation. Nor can I recall a single *puerperal sepsis* developing as a result of a home confinement. I can only assume that these hardy women had become immune to the germs of their environment. Very possibly, had they gone into hospital for their confinement a number of them would have developed infections to which they had no immunity.

Because ideas familiar now were not available to us then, we made mistakes. We kept women in bed for two weeks after a birth, which was too long. Many developed trouble walking and had pain in their feet from lack of exercise.

And there is a case I recall of a young attractive newly-wed mother whose first baby was stillborn and so deformed it was classified as a monster. In a year there was a second one, and that was followed by a third—all monsters. At the woman's request, we sterilized her, not realizing until years later the possible error. We assumed that she was at fault. Today we know that there was at least a fifty-fifty chance that all she needed was a change of husbands.

A word about my business methods. I early evolved a method of keeping records that was in the long run moderately efficient. It was based on what I think was called the McCaskey book-keeping system, with its set of special forms for recording patients' findings and their financial status. Each weekend I added up the week's business and recorded it under six columns as follows.

1	2	3	4	5	6
Date	Cash Business	Credit Business	Total Business (2 + 3)	Paid on Account	Total Cash (2 + 5)

From these weekly reports it was very easy to total the figures for every month and year of practice.

The records show that cash receipts of my first month's practice were $68.40, the first five months $668.40 and the first year $1,872.90. As can be seen, the financial returns from medical services were somewhat uncertain. After meeting payments on the house, travel and office expenses, this allowed for only lean living. A doctor in a new locality got rather more than his share of the "slow pay" and the "poor pay". However, this income was in line with the belief held then that it took a family doctor about three years to reach a reasonable livable income. To own a house, car and summer cottage took a lifetime's work. I was collecting from 80 to 85 per cent of my fees, having learned early in my experience to render an account promptly when requested. If I did so, it would often be paid at once. On the other hand, if I had to mail the account, it might be many months before the bill was paid. This required that my books be kept up-to-date. After some years I adopted the plan of suing two or three people annually by putting their accounts into the local village court for collection. These were always people who owed me a substantial amount, who were ignoring me by going to another physician, and whom I was sure were able to pay. I wished the public to know that I expected to be remunerated for my services. It is interesting that at least half of those sued in this manner promptly returned as patients. Needless to say, I preferred my own efforts at collecting to those of professional bill collectors, because I thought I could get better results and with less annoyance to the patients.

In that first decade of practice before the wonders of modern surgery we struggled with many problems.

Colin was a tall lean man of seventy when he started coming to me for a soft rubber catheter, and he continued coming at six-month intervals, being unable to void without using such a device. He carried the catheter everywhere with him in the top of his hat, curled up in a piece of old newspaper, and used it without any attempt whatever at cleanliness. His urine, loaded with infection, looked like milk. It was a revelation to see a man living in apparent good health in this manner. I was taught that a man living a "catheter life" was quite ill and hadn't long to live—a maximum of perhaps three years. But Colin went merrily along for another eight years, when he died after a brief bout with pneumonia.

Men rarely are seen today living with dependence on a catheter. Urinary tract surgery is now one of surgical medicine's greatest gifts to mankind. Although in the twenties creditable techniques in urinary surgery had been perfected, surgeons were having some difficulty proving the worth of such operations to the public and to other doctors because they were so new. It takes a few years to popularize any major surgical procedure. Also, it seems that men and women tend to feel instinctively that there is something sacred about their procreative organs with their *adnexa*. Judging the basement apartment with its plumbing to be at least as important as the upper storey, they have been hesitant to permit tampering with these areas until convinced that any surgical interference will surely be permanently helpful.

MacPherson, who suffered from early prostatism, a common affliction of elderly men, was typical of his kind. Nearing seventy, it was his custom every few weeks to have several cronies in for an evening beer party. Without fail, about 4 a.m. the next morning the bell in my surgery would ring. Mac would first apologize for bothering me and then rather shamefacedly ask for relief with a catheter. I would accommodate him and repeat the procedure twice a day for two or three days thereafter—when he would be fully restored until the next drinking bout. He refused surgery for three years, until a time came when I could no longer bring his voiding back to normal.

Mac helped to teach me what it took several years to learn—that it was best with these patients to insist upon surgery after the first catheterization, because further use of the catheter so often gave only temporary relief. Moreover, the earlier the surgeon took over, the better were the patient's prospects for full recovery.

Jerry's was a rare case and it too taught me a lot. An Irishman and a farmer, after thirty years of hard work and careful saving he had put together an estate of four hundred acres, built a new barn and house. This was when disaster struck. He could no longer swallow any food. When he asked me to take over his health at this time, he was more than a patient, he was a friend, as he had been our closest neighbor when I was a boy at home. A careful history and an initial examination in a city hospital under the direction of a consultant revealed this story.

In his teens Jerry had had pneumonia accompanied by pleurisy with empyema, i.e., pus in his chest. For some unknown reason the doctor did not drain this but waited until it burst through the chest wall and drained itself. As a result of such prolonged neglect of an extensive inflammation, Jerry's gullet was eventually drawn to one side and contracted so that food couldn't pass down it. To help him in swallowing, I was advised to get a set of oesophageal dilators of different sizes and use them in succession, starting with the smaller ones.

I didn't relish the task of passing the dilators down his gullet, having had no training in this rather rare procedure; it would be very easy to push one through the gullet wall. Fortunately, there was no such accident, and the use of the dilators every few months gave Jerry considerable temporary relief. During this time he lived largely on soups, milk mixtures and syrups, dying some four years later from bronchial pneumonia. In fact, he had starved to death. Today all patients with empyema have the purulent material drained by cutting away a section of a rib—a simple and common procedure. Jerry's experience probably indicates that in olden times people frequently recovered from empyema by waiting until it burst through their chest wall.

Another unusual case comes to mind that invites comparison with procedures of the present time. Roderick's stomach ulcer had troubled him off and on for thirty years, for relief of which —so he maintained—he had taken several barrels of baking soda. When I saw him he presented a picture which must be rare today. The upper part of his belly was greatly enlarged, and he couldn't eat enough to keep him alive.

Washing out his stomach produced a surprising quantity of fluid and his abdomen flattened out. The ulcer was located at the outlet of his stomach and the inflammation accompanying it over many years had gradually closed this exit passage. Food that could not pass simply collected in his stomach. Roderick was shown how to wash out his own stomach, and by doing this daily for a couple of weeks he got relief. On several occasions he was put to bed for ten days or so and fed only liquids with a 50 cc syringe through a small rubber duodenal tube—and this also helped. This small tube was swallowed until the lower end went beyond the stomach so that the food given him bypassed the ulcer, permitting partial healing. However, in spite of all such measures, Roderick eventually had to submit to major surgery—and with good results.

Surgeons of the twenties were having admirable success in operating for this ailment. The usual procedure was to make a new stomach opening and connect it to the bowel. But though this method worked satisfactorily, surgeons were to learn a few years later that it was preferable as well to remove a liberal portion of the stomach.

Acute appendicitis was a problem then as it is now. But there was a difference. Then we saw a much higher percentage of patients who had been suffering from the affliction for a week or more. A number of older physicians and a few of the younger ones believed it best to subject the patient to several days of starvation before resorting to surgery. There was considerable justification for this belief as quite a number of such patients did recover without an operation. However, there were dangers in waiting for those few days which gave the inflamed appendix time to bury itself in a mass of irritated tissue, and this called for skillful dissection if it had to be removed later. Furthermore, some patients went on to widespread abdominal inflammation and death.

There were unusual situations involving the appendix with which we weren't very familiar. I recall one tragedy. A leading business man in our community developed appendicitis and died in a London hospital. My consultant and I had been slow in diagnosing the trouble because the appendix was far back near a kidney and the symptoms were not the common ones.

Tena's case was unusual but the outcome was happier. A girl of eighteen, she had been ill ten days under the care of a physician who believed in a trial of starvation. He was not available when I saw her for the first time late one evening in her home seven miles from the village. She had a mass in her abdomen as large as an orange. It was obviously an abscess caused by appendicitis and it needed draining. This was not a particularly difficult procedure, but I didn't have the courage to do it unaided in the home. I preferred to have it done in hospital. The problem was that a three-day blizzard was raging and I had had difficulty getting even the seven miles to her home over snow-blocked roads. To take her to hospital at night, a distance of ten miles, in a sleigh behind a team of horses plunging through snow drifts would be very trying for her. Also, the abscess had been there for a number of days and seemed to be well walled off. Waiting another twenty-four hours didn't appear to be risking very much. So I planned taking her to hospital the next morning.

When I returned the next day Tena's abdomen was as flat as a pie plate. I couldn't believe what I saw until the mother showed me a basin filled with purulent material she had passed. Nature had healed the abscess by draining it through the bowel. In another four days Tena was up and about. Nature has more ways than one of getting us better—sometimes. There is no lesson to be drawn from this as it was the only time I saw an abscess from appendicitis drained in this way.

III. Before the Age of Miracles: A Different and Distant World

I shall never forget our first Christmas in Lucknow. It was a dismal occasion. On Christmas Eve a blizzard started and shortly after noon on Christmas Day I left by horse and cutter for a farm home where there were two boys with a rash, fever, sore throat and discharging ears—symptoms of the dreaded scarlet fever. It was my first visit to them. The concession roads were impassable; I made my way along poorly marked trails over fields and through woods, travelling at least twice the distance a crow would have taken to cover the five miles.

When I arrived home at eight that evening it was to find my wife Marjorie sitting on the stairs weeping. Her day had been dreary, the Christmas dinner was ruined. However, she was naturally of a cheerful disposition and soon her gloom disappeared. Her final word on the day was: "Once I said I would go with you anywhere, even to the North Pole if necessary, and now I think I damn near have."

My wife with her kindness and understanding of people was of marvellous assistance to me. On one occasion a woman presented herself at the office in such precipitate labor that Marjorie offered her our bedroom and provided her with all nursing care until she and the babe left in ten days for home. It was a measure of her understanding that she purposely obtained little information about my patients so that when a close friend asked how so-and-so was she could truthfully say she didn't know. This was a significant contribution to my work because most people dislike their illnesses and health shortcomings discussed unless by themselves. I soon found that my wife was a stellar helpmate in facing the health problems of the community.

Personal relations are important in the medical profession as elsewhere, and not just the relationship between doctor and patient. When I came to Lucknow, it had three physicians and really didn't need a fourth. Dr. William Connell was a young man like myself with whom I was to have innumerable pleasant and helpful associations. The second, an elderly man who derived most of his income from a drug store, didn't delay long in confiding that it was most ungentlemanly, to say the least, for me to settle in the community. The third had been an able family doctor before he became addicted to alcohol, and he could at times make my life very frustrating, though he was friendly and affable on social occasions and when ill called on me to attend him. One of his most exasperating habits was to ridicule my treatment of patients in their presence and throw out from patients' homes all medicine prescribed by me and other doctors. To one of my patients he declared that the harmless boracic acid solution used as an eye lotion would destroy his vision. In time, when this colleague became an advanced or confirmed alcoholic, he joined the club of "life-saver doctors"—as we derisively called them—as one means of recovering his lost practice. Such doctors were wont to tell their patients, "You have come to me just in time," or, "A few more days' delay in coming to me would have been too late." The more zealous of these practitioners sometimes were known as "before-breakfast life savers."

This attitude of doctors discrediting their fellow practitioners was the exception, but far from rare in the 1920's and 1930's. Most of my confrères were helpful and some exceedingly so.

I cannot overlook the help given me by a Goderich doctor, Dr. Harold Taylor, who was certified in both radiology and surgery. He was one of the wisest doctors I have been privileged to meet, an excellent diagnostician and very careful in treatment. I remember one of his dictums, "Don't use a forceps in confinements until prepared to walk two miles to get them."

To my knowledge, the first doctor in Ontario to take a partner was a Dr. McMillan of Grimsby, in 1930, but there must have been earlier ones. It was in that year that my colleagues and I tried an experiment in cooperation. About eight family doctors from different communities got together and decided on a kind of specialization, using the facilities of Wingham General Hospital, the nearest one to me. It was arranged between us that two of our number would do most of the surgery and one would become skilled in pinning hips—that is, in treating the common hip fracture; two others would give anaesthetics, and I would increase my knowledge of cardiology and do electrocardiograms. This arrangement persisted for some years, until specialization became a common practice. Our group was large enough to give me considerable experience with heart ailments.

One bizarre occurrence comes to mind as a result of this pooling of skills. Dr. Connell phoned at five a.m. one cold winter morning from Wingham Hospital to say: "I have a man of forty-five with a perforated stomach ulcer. While taking him on the elevator to the operating room it seemed to me he looked more like a person with a heart attack. Will you come over and tell me what you think?"

In explanation, a perforated ulcer is one that has eaten through the stomach wall and calls for emergency closure. The electrocardiogram tracing in this case showed that the man did indeed have an acute coronary attack. He was, in short, desperately ill with two lethal conditions, a heart attack and a perforated stomach ulcer. How could his life be saved?

I pointed out to Dr. Connell that recent literature indicated that some ulcer holes would heal if the patient was fed a light milk diet through a duodenal tube. With this treatment perhaps surgery could be delayed for a day or so.

But Dr. Connell rejected this temporizing policy and decided to operate at once. "If he should die without my closing that hole I would never forgive myself," he said.

The patient lived for only two days. In spite of the fatal outcome, I had the highest respect for Dr. Connell's judgment. It was his decision; I was only a consultant on the case. But whatever else we were on that cold winter morning—we were two pretty lonely general practitioners. I remember that part clearly.

A certain daily routine, allowing flexibility, was essential and with the passage of time my working life settled into a recognizable pattern. From Monday to Saturday inclusive I spent the mornings making house calls and hospital visits; the afternoons and evenings I spent in the office. Invariably there were ten to fifteen patients in hospital. Sundays I would catch up by making calls I had been forced to overlook or delay, and by writing up the office accounts and patients' histories.

Had I to do it over again, I would not have home and office in the same building, though there was one distinct advantage: I didn't have far to go when someone called at the office at night—usually the victim of an accident. Although part of the house, the office had its own entrance. It consisted of a waiting room, an examining room and a dispensary with running water and a bench for limited laboratory equipment, including a microscope.

Night visits were never an extensive part of my practice. They were more frequent in the very early years when there might be two or three or possibly four a week. As my practice grew, night work decreased due to the reasonableness of the younger patients, who learned to trust my judgment as to the urgency of their condition. If I advised waiting till morning to see me, they usually would. It was much harder to get similar cooperation from the elderly, some of whom seemed to think I was under an obligation to be at their beck and call.

There was Sandy, for instance, a tall, thin, dried-out man of sixty-five. He complained over the phone so effectively of a "headache" that I felt he might be having a brain hemorrhage. It was six in the evening, in the midst of the winter's worst blizzard. On my way to his home, while facing the bitter snow-laden wind, I lost the road several times and found myself travelling close to the rail fence. Arriving at his place, I stabled the horse and by pounding on the door roused Sandy from a sound sleep. His toothache was better. I concluded he had an abscessed tooth root well back in an upper jaw. And he just hadn't bothered to phone that I wasn't needed. I had trouble forgiving him during the following two weeks while the frozen skin peeled off my cheeks. It reminded me of a Russian saying, "Not even a philosopher can bear a toothache calmly."

Somewhat later in my career, I had another unusual tooth case. Henry's sister phoned rather frantically one morning that her brother had lost his lower plate of false teeth and was so upset she didn't know what to do. I had been Henry's doctor for ten years. He was a tall thin man of a gentlemanly type, deliberate in speech and movements. He wasn't the kind of person to get easily excited or upset and I couldn't imagine why he wanted me rather than a neighbor or his brother who lived close by.

I found him in his bedroom in the upstairs of his frame farm house searching everywhere for his teeth. I felt a bit silly joining in a further search while we took the bed clothes apart at least three times, looked through the other room furniture and everywhere on the floor. Then suddenly I thought, "Why not look in the most obvious place, down his throat?" Sure enough, with a light and mirror I could see the plate sitting down there and could just touch it with the tip of my finger. A call to the local dentist brought him out with a hooked wire and with his long fingers he lifted out the plate.

"Henry, may I take the plate to my office for a day as I would like to make a drawing of it and measure it?"

"Take it and keep it—I will never use it again." And he didn't. When he died suddenly six or seven years later, the undertaker suggested I return the teeth.

On looking up the literature I found that partial plates or broken ones are frequently swallowed but uncommonly a whole plate. In elderly people the throat muscles become very relaxed and insensitive.

Henry's plate measured 3¼ inches at its widest. If not removed, it would have caused early swelling and death soon, possibly in three or four days.

Another amusing incident happened one New Year's eve at 11 p.m. My wife Marjorie and I were about to leave for a party to celebrate the advent of the New Year when the office bell rang. To say the least, it was annoying to be summoned to work at such a time. In the waiting room a friend greeted me, "I have cut myself on my bottom."

While he leaned over my surgery table I put three stitches into an inch long cut on his hip. He didn't need any anaesthetic, as he already had started to celebrate the New Year.

"How did you do this?"

"I bit myself."

"Don't be ridiculous."

"That is my story and I am sticking to it."

He went on his way. I thought that he was merely trying to make amends for his untimely visit by amusing me. Four days later he came in for removal of the sutures.

"Are you going to tell me the truth today about the accident."

"I bit myself; that is my story and I'm sticking to it. My new false teeth were bothering me. They were in my hip pocket when I fell on the icy sidewalk."

Transportation

How explain what transportation was like in the twenties, especially nights and during winter, in those days before lighted macadam highways and road crews with high-powered equipment to clear them? We doctors were not complainers for the most part, but as one classmate—Dr. George Case—put it, writing from Manitoulin Island in one of the snow belt areas: "Watching a horse's tail bob up and down for mile after mile through pitch holes would be hell if one didn't like treating sick people."

We in the Lucknow district were also in a so-called snow belt. The gravel roads were adequate for travel with my Model T

Ford (a touring model cost $385 in 1924, a sedan $685) except in winter and for a two-or-three-week muddy period in spring. Winters were often drawn-out sieges of stinging cold from Hallowe'en to Easter, punctuated with an occasional three-day blizzard.

In the late fall we would begin to fight the snow and ice with shovels, tire chains which needed constant repair, and a box of sand in the car trunk, the weight of which gave traction to the rear wheels; we used to sprinkle the sand in front of the wheels when stalled on ice. We always carried a heavy logging chain in the event we needed a pull from a passing team of horses. The cars were unheated and we dressed as for the outside weather. Then around the seventh of December we gave up the struggle between snow and car and jacked the latter up on blocks in the garage. From then on we used the horse and cutter.

I always had two horses, and one winter owned a third. They were tended by an hostler, but I drove myself. My mainstay was a sorrel mare which could travel at a steady ten-mile-an-hour clip. She wasn't very intelligent as she didn't know enough to slow to a walk on going up a hill unless I reined her in. And whenever she entered the village on returning from a trip, no matter how tired she was, away she would dash with her tail in the air. Someone had taught her this. Another horse, a huge black brute, could also travel fast, but was a bit demented. On being hitched to the cutter, he would rear up, plunge backward a few feet and then dash ahead. It was too bad if I wasn't in the cutter ready for these antics. I did not know about this quirk when I bought him. I found out later that it was advisable to hitch him close to and facing a building. In this way he had first to swing around, and by that time he had forgotten his usual starting maneuvers—but there wasn't always a building available.

The cutter was as comfortable as I could make it, with a top closed in on the back and a side door. An old Ford car light on the dash sustained by a tank of carbide under the seat cast a beam about a hundred feet ahead. A buffalo robe and a lantern under it for warmth completed the equipment, along with my fur coat and gauntlets. All would go well until the cutter upset, which happened frequently, and this sometimes would demolish the top. Once I was upset so quickly and unexpectedly that the mare ran away. Before she was stopped she had kicked the cutter apart, and I rode home seated on a pile of fragments. Many a day I drove fifty miles, and on one occasion a hundred miles—using three horses in relay.

It is too bad we didn't have skidoos. There were snowmobiles on the market—big powerful machines on large caterpillar treads and skis. They cost about $700 and consumed gasoline at the rate of a gallon every seven miles. Some doctors tried them but reported that to steer one of the monsters was so tiring that a twenty-mile journey would leave the driver exhausted.

From a financial point of view, winter practice was very unsatisfactory. It was hopeless to expect to earn a reasonable income. On many days we did not attend enough patients to make ends meet. A trip ten miles distant would take most of a morning. There was little time to spare for the office. The fees were regulated by the official fee schedule, by what the patient could pay and by the charges of older physicians, which in some instances were ridiculously low—such as two dollars for a ten-mile trip. My fees were two dollars for a visit in and near the village, five to ten dollars for a distance of six to ten miles. Fortunately, it didn't cost much to maintain a horse—less than twenty-five cents a day for feed.

Who were the men who chose such a life as this? At one time we made a survey of the fifty or so doctors of Huron County, which is mostly rural, and found that about half came from villages and the countryside, the other half from cities. I have never been convinced that country-bred doctors tend to choose country practice and city boys stay by preference in the cities, as has been often contended.

Progress in transportation came slowly. Although car starters were invented in 1913, people continued to crank cars in the

1920's and well into the 1930's. In consequence, we treated many wrist fractures from back-firing. Snow-plowing equipment came into use in many parts of Ontario about 1930 but not in the Lucknow area until late in that decade, when it began as a political issue. Why waste money this way? was the general feeling. However, when once people had a taste of plowed roads travel by horse and cutter disappeared like magic; in as short a time as two years automobiles took over all roads, even those in remote rural areas.

While conditions of travel made all the difference between comfort and discomfort in the performance of his duties, a doctor's first concern, then as now, was the patient and his own skill in making use of available drugs. One has only to look back to the early twenties to see how far medical science has progressed in our time.

In the office we dispensed all the common tablets, powders, ointments and liquid preparations judged to be helpful, and occasionally wrote prescriptions for the rarer products to be filled by one of the two local pharmacists. We had numerous inexpensive and "shot-gun" mixtures, so called because of their many ingredients, which were given for stomach upsets, coughs or as tonics. Morphine, aspirin, digitalis and Luminal—or phenobarbital, to use its correct name—were indispensable. The latter was discovered in 1912 and remains to this day one of the most useful tranquilizers. I bought Luminal tablets in five-thousand lots every few months. Though I looked carefully for them, I never recognized a barbiturate addict in my practice. One patient who comes to mind took five grains three times a day for months and then desisted for a month over a period of thirty years. He was a tense and highly excitable person, but the use of Luminal quieted him and helped keep his blood pressure within reasonable limits, contributing to his longevity of 94 years. He insisted that he never developed an abnormal craving for the drug.

There is probably no counting the people who watched helplessly while a relative or friend died slowly of diabetes before the discovery of insulin in 1921. Likewise, a perforated appendix was often fatal. Pernicious anemia was a death sentence. One in four pneumonia patients died. And because tuberculosis was diagnosed late, it resulted often in certain death, frequently after long periods in sanatoria.

The handful of synthetic drugs we found useful included:

Arsenic	Chloral Hydrate	Mercury
Alcohol	Chloroform	Paraldehyde
Apomorphine	Digitalis	Quinine
Aspirin	Ether	Salicylic Acid
Barbiturates	Heroin	Salvarsan
Benzoic Acid	Iron	Sassafras
Carbolic Acid	Morphine	

Let us look at a few of these. Two had specific effects on disease, namely quinine in malaria and digitalis in heart ailments. Two others, aspirin and the barbiturates, although not in the life-saving class, conferred untold benefits on ailing mankind. But strange to say, only one of these drugs could halt a deadly infection—that is, Salvarsan for syphilis.

Paracelsus of the sixteenth century recommended arsenic for syphilis. However, it wasn't widely used until 1910 when Paul Ehrlich announced an arsenical compound known as Salvarsan, or 606, as a cure for the disease.

Paul Ehrlich (1854-1915) laid the foundation for the coming age of chemotherapy which began in the early 1930's. His work was initially inspired by that of Robert Koch, who identified the tubercle bacillus but never succeeded in finding a means of destroying it. Ehrlich noticed that the cells and parts of the cells of the body tissues took selective staining with dyes and he conceived the idea that dyes might be used to deliver a chemical to the part of the body where it was required. With an eye on the spirochete causing syphilis, he chose experiments with arsenic compounds. In 1909, after painstakingly investigating many substances for several years, he came up with two compounds which showed fair results in animals. Finally, when the list of substances reached 606, a highly effective and apparently non-toxic substance proved to be the answer. Eventually, it was called Salvarsan, or 606. It attacked the spirochete of syphilis without harming the host.

Arsenic was popularly used also as a back-up medicine to iron for anemia.

There are several accounts of events which led to the discovery of aspirin. One is that in the 1890's a chemist employed in the Bayer Laboratories sought something to ease the pain of his father's arthritis. He found it in an almost forgotten compound which had been made some forty years earlier—acetylsalicylic acid. Bayer purified, tested and marketed it in 1899 as aspirin.

From the start aspirin, a mild analgesic and antipyretic, was a great commercial success. Enormous quantities are sold over the counter today in every country in the world. It is still the most widely used medicine for aches and pains and for reducing fever.

Barbituric acid was developed a few years later, i.e., early in this century, by the German pharmaceutical industry. It was a white crystalline organic compound which by modification yielded the barbiturates. There is now a whole family of barbiturates. Its most common preparations are phenobarbital (Luminal), amobarbital (Amytal), pentobarbital (Nembutal) and secobarbital (Seconal). In medical practice barbiturates are used to treat insomnia, anxiety, nervous tension and epilepsy. Barbiturates are popular as drugs of abuse among people who want to experience effects similar to those produced by large doses of alcohol, such as euphoria and temporary relief from daily worries and anxieties.

The first barbiturate was Veronal (barbital sodium)—a long-acting one. Luminal followed soon after and—as I have said—was popular in the 1920's. Its effects did not last as long as those of Veronal. Of course, Luminal didn't mix with alcohol safely. Taken with alcohol, the barbiturates often give unpredictable and dangerous results. I recall a young lawyer who on a worrisome day took a Seconal tablet at noon, followed by a couple of stiff drinks of rum. After a sleep, he was shocked because he couldn't remember any of the day's events, including a business contract he had signed.

It is rather a whimsical notion to include sassafras, which comes from a member of the laurel family of North American trees, in the list of useful drugs. Its scope of usefulness was limited. The usual treatment for head lice was to tie tightly around the head towels and cloths soaked in coal oil, but some doctors preferred to use a solution made from the aromatic bark or foliage of the sassafras tree. I had no experience with it, but was told it made an evil-smelling head bandage.

In the decade before the revolution in therapeutic medicine I was seeing several new patients each year with the full-blown picture of pernicious anemia. They presented a striking appearance with their pale lemon-yellow skin. A disease of mid-life and always a death sentence, pernicious anemia was twice as common in men as in women. I had a slight personal interest in it as my paternal grandfather died of it in 1910, when he was in his early forties. It tended to run in families. One authority lists the occurrence in six successive generations of the same family.

The victims of this disease were often easily recognized for exhaustion, in addition to their dry yellow scruffy skin, gave them away. Weariness and languor had come on so slowly and insidiously they couldn't give a precise date to its beginning. In spite of it, surprisingly, they had lost little weight and were still eating quite well. Numbness and tingling of the fingers and toes were common along with some numbness of the nose. Answers to questions would reveal a dry mouth and a burning sore tongue.

To confirm the diagnosis, we studied a thin smear of blood on a glass slide under a microscope, estimated the hemoglobin, and counted the red blood cells. The percentage of hemoglobin bore a special relationship to the percentage of red blood cells present. The blood film in many instances showed the typical text-book picture of this type of anemia, but not always if there was only a slight abnormality. When in doubt, we often passed a small tube into the stomach, obtained some contents which should show an absence of stomach acid. But to me this test was unreliable, and time proved me right. I didn't know then what is generally recognized now, that as many as 15 per cent of people forty to sixty years of age have no stomach acid, and this percentage is even greater in older folk. There was another reason for unreliability: diarrhea and quick stomach-emptying time are now known to result sometimes in a loss of stomach acid.

Most of the patients had both a loss of vibration sense and a loss of position sense in their limbs, with a tendency to stumble. The loss of feeling in their fingers and toes would slowly extend upwards.

In arriving at a diagnosis we had to think of the possibility of other severe anemias such as that from the rare infestation with a tapeworm, the occasional non-tropical sprue, and the nutritional anemias. For instance, some food fads lacking the protein of meats, eggs, and milk bring on a severe anemia. A folic-acid deficiency had to be considered. Also, cancer, particularly that of the stomach.

In treatment, we urged a liberal diet of the best foods and gave a mixture of iron and arsenic in the form of Fowler's Solution—starting with three drops three times a day and increasing the dose daily by one drop until nausea came on. This usually occurred when the dose reached eleven drops three times a day. Often dilute hydrochloric acid was added to the meals to make up for the lack of stomach acid. In terminal stages, blood transfusions might be resorted to.

Pernicious anemia was a chronic malady with remarkable remissions at unpredictable intervals, during which time patients could feel quite well and return to work for several months, even as long as three years. The number of remissions varied from two to five or six and they were always followed by a return of the severe anemia, or crises; often the patient died during the third such crisis. The disease had been called a leisure-killer, taking as long as five years to claim its victim.

It was in 1926 that Dr. George Richard Minot of the Harvard Medical School and Dr. William Parry Murphy of Peter Bent Brigham Hospital announced the life-saving properties of liver for these patients. For medical science this was a stunning victory and the story of how it all came about is remarkable.*

Two years before this, in 1924, Dr. George H. Whipple, a pathologist and head of the New Hooper Foundation, the research department of the University of California's Medical School, had started a study of the disease. It was already known at that time that all anemias are characterized by a decrease in the red blood cells carrying oxygen to our tissues. In health we have about five million red cells per cubic millimeter in our blood. With pernicious anemia these may drop to as few as five hundred thousand, when the blood will look little better than colored water. Healthy red cells live about twenty days, and when they die must be replaced at the rate of millions per second. In the light of these facts, Dr. Whipple experimented with dogs. First he produced artificial anemia by drawing off blood until the number of red cells was down to 50 per cent of normal. Then he devised and fed the animals diets to provide essential nourishment to maintain life but lacking blood-building properties. Next, over a period of many months, he tried various supplementary foods that might hasten the production of red cells: milk, eggs, lettuce, a variety of meats. When liver was administered, the results were almost unbelievable. In as short a time as two weeks the red-cell content of the blood was restored to normal.

Hearing of this work with dogs, Dr. Minot enlisted the help of Dr. Murphy and together they experimented to discover whether Dr. Whipple's findings held true with human beings.

* George H. Whipple, M.D., "The Disease That Always Killed," *The Reader's Digest*, November 1971.

They stuffed their pernicious anemia patients with all the liver they would take. When a group numbering forty-five had with one exception responded by a return to normalcy, Dr. Minot read a paper before a medical meeting on May 4, 1926, that received world-wide attention.

Immediately, practicing doctors everywhere began feeding their anemia patients raw liver. Soon powdered liver appeared on the market, followed in 1931 by an injectable liver extract 400,000 times as potent. And in 1934 Doctors Whipple, Minot and Murphy were accorded medicine's highest honor—the Nobel Prize.

It was twenty years after Dr. Minot read his electrifying paper before the anti-pernicious anemia factor in liver was identified and a compound known as vitamin B_{12} (see Chapter VIII) became available as a convenient and inexpensive therapy having everything necessary in minute quantities to control this disease. In the meantime, to doctors practicing in the twenties and thirties it seemed a miracle for dying patients to become new people after a liver diet of several weeks. It was amusing to note with what pleasure they reported that the first evidence of improvement was a return of feeling to the tip of their nose. If there was no improvement within three weeks, we looked for another explanation for the anemia. This became a therapeutic test. We soon learned that after dosages of liver for even a day or two it became impossible to diagnose this type of anemia from the blood, such profound changes take place so quickly after liver is introduced to the body.

Liver therapy for pernicious anemia was one of the first of today's miracle drugs. It not only gave these people back good health, but sustained them in good health for many years.

It was my good fortune that insulin was known and available when I started practice. Sir Frederick Banting and Dr. Charles Best of Toronto in May 1921 made their remarkable discovery of its value in the treatment of diabetes. At that time this disease with its punishing symptoms of a ravenous hunger and thirst was sometimes called the sugar sickness. Commercial insulin was made available in limited quantities to practicing doctors late in 1923 by Connaught Medical Research Laboratories, Toronto.

I recall only one diabetic patient of pre-insulin days, a charming vivacious country girl of fourteen who was losing weight steadily. After being put on the limited diabetic diet of that day she seemed to waste away faster than ever, and eventually died. This was in 1924. I say this patient was pre-insulin because for some reason, I do not recollect, I did not use insulin; probably I couldn't get it.

The "merry" month of May annually ushers in our summer. But May 1927 was a gloomy one for me. I lost three pneumonia patients in that month, a record so depressing that it made me think of leaving medicine. But I had nowhere to go; I had no training in anything else. The tragedy was that each victim was a young father with a family of small children.

Doctors recognize two types of pneumonia: lobar and bronchial. One of our lungs has two large parts or lobes, the other has three lobes. In lobar pneumonia the lung infection involves a whole lobe or lobes, which become airless and solid. Bronchial pneumonia occurs when the infection involves numerous scattered small parts of one or both lungs.

These types are easily distinguished on chest examination. In my training days in hospitals the pneumonia patients we saw were chiefly of the lobar type. This type persisted in my practice until about 1930 when, for some unaccountable reason, it disappeared—and for years thereafter I encountered only patients with bronchial pneumonia. Doctors in the Toronto area say this was not true there, but it certainly applied to the counties of Huron and Bruce.

Each of the three patients who died in May 1927 had lobar pneumonia. One died with a complication of meningitis (inflammation of the brain lining), the second had peritonitis (inflammation of the lining of the abdomen), and the third had a most unexpected and uncommon ending from a disaster I didn't know might occur. At one of my daily morning visits to his home the competent nurse in charge showed me a basin full of blood which the patient had passed by bowel in the night. Her quizzical expression and comments showed that she had doubts about my diagnosis. She was thinking that perhaps my patient had typhoid fever, but I knew this couldn't be. However, as a precaution I obtained a sample of blood for submission to the Department of Health in Toronto for testing, then rushed home to consult my textbooks. Sure enough, one authority noted that massive bowel hemorrhage could be a complication of a severe pneumonia.

The treatment of pneumonia in those days consisted of supportive measures: rest in bed, good food, lots of liquids, sponging for sweating, mustard and linseed plasters with aspirin for chest pain, fluids by rectum for patients not drinking enough, and hypnotics if necessary to ensure sleep. One of the elderly and highly competent physicians in Toronto believed the best thing he could do for pneumonia patients was to give them enough morphine repeatedly to ensure that they were resting and always free of the anxiety and apprehension accompanying this disease. There was much to be said for this therapy.

Everyone, doctor and members of the family, anxiously awaited the crisis marking the turning point of this disease, that dramatic moment when the resources of the patient finally overcame the poisons of the infecting germs. The patient would suddenly start breathing quietly, stop sweating, probably turn over in bed, ask for a drink of water and go to sleep. On seeing this, an experienced doctor wouldn't need to use his thermometer; he would know that the temperature was normal again.

All this was changed by the mass production of penicillin in 1945. True, in 1928 Sir Alexander Fleming, a bacteriologist of St. Mary's Hospital, London, England, noticed that a mold of unknown substance apparently destroyed staphylococcus germs on a culture plate, and named the mold penicillin. He suggested that it might be useful in treating infections. But it was ignored for a dozen years, until England was fighting for survival in World War II. We will pick up that story later in Chapter VIII.

The problems of tuberculosis, like those of pneumonia, were different from the problems of today and one case I recall vividly was that of Curly, a tall handsome young man, one of the brightest and a good friend. After graduation from normal school he was hired as a teacher in a country school where he put into practice his own advanced ideas of education. Each morning the whole school spent an hour discussing current news from his copy of the Toronto daily paper. Should the school program drag at any time, he might bundle the children into his car and take them on a sight-seeing tour of the countryside. These progressive ideas shocked the school board and he was promptly fired.

Curly was about thirty years old when he became ill with a cough, night sweats, flushing of the face and loss of weight—pulmonary tuberculosis. In his childhood his mother had died of tuberculosis meningitis. Curly was put to bed on the porch of his home and the windows were kept open at all times, following the approved treatment of the day. After a wintery blizzard the bed clothes would be covered with snow. He died in less than two years and I can never forget how keenly he felt that life was cheating him.

And there were Tom and Margaret of my village, a brother and sister who died in their early twenties, probably having contracted the disease from their father, a McGill University professor, who followed them a few years later.

These three young victims of the tuberculosis scourge were representative of those I encountered with this disease in the 1920's—that is, nearly all were in their late teens or twenties, and they didn't live long, two or three years. They were said to have consumption, a word coined because the disease seemed to consume the whole body; sometimes it was called galloping consumption, to indicate the speed with which it carried off its victims.

The disease was well advanced when discovered because there were so few diagnostic facilities. There were no tubercular skin testings or mass chest X-ray programs, and few hospitals were prepared to X-ray the chest and interpret the film. Physical examination of the patient was usually inconclusive. The symptoms were cough, pain in the chest, night sweats, loss of weight and often euphoria. As stated, the treatment was rest in bed and fresh air; the rest did the good and not the cold air. The disease was hard to control because there was a large pool of infection about and no effective drugs. For those who could afford it there might be a visit to Arizona. Some were referred to a sanatorium, but for years sanatorium beds were at a premium. Treatment there was a long-stay proposition, usually from two to ten years and even for life. It was a mysterious disease, with much debate at that time whether it was an endogenous or exogenous infection—that is, whether it came from within the patient or from outside. This indicates how far we have now progressed in understanding.

Even at that time surgeons were doing useful work in controlling the disease. They had learned that putting the lung at rest helped in recovery. This they did in several ways. As early as 1900 they devised a way of immobilizing or splinting the lung by putting air in the pleural cavity around it; this was called the pneumothorax procedure. It was popular by 1920 and proved to be a very marked advance in treatment. Pneumoperitoneum was another method used, the injection of air into the peritonal cavity which reduced the respiratory activity of the lung. Crushing the phrenic nerve had the same effect. Then in the 1920's thoracoplasty—removal of several ribs to produce permanent collapse of the lung—became a treatment for selective patients, usually those with only one lung involved.

In 1924 the Ontario Government began to take an interest in this problem disease by adding a Tuberculosis Section to the Division of Infectious Disease Control. In the same year, Dr. G. C. Brink introduced a mobile chest X-ray service, the first in the world. This expanded rapidly and soon a specialized service covering both diagnosis and treatment was visualized. As a result, late in the decade and early in the 1930's tuberculosis control began to separate itself from the mainstream of medicine. Because of the highly infectious nature of the disease the general practitioner was unable to control it effectively and it became a specialized field with specialists in charge. This development led to a change in medical school teaching: students were instructed to diagnose the illness, then refer the patient to special facilities.

All of this heralded other later advances—the compulsory pasteurization of milk, the drive for funds for research through the sale of Christmas seals.

We take the wonder drugs so for granted these days that it is difficult to appreciate the vast changes they have brought about in medical therapy affecting our daily life. The following is a homely incident common in the era before antibiotics.

Mrs. Annie J. consulted me about the end of a finger swollen and painful. There was a small break in the skin, obviously an infection from a skin abrasion, which in turn was the result of an accident while changing a car tire. Though it was a small wound, I knew it could be serious, that infections from the soil were often very virulent and even deadly. And so it proved; the germs steadily forged ahead into the soft tissues of this woman's fingers and hand. It was six months' treatment at home and in hospital with bathing in hot antiseptic solutions and various dressings before the infection was checked or died out. By that time not much remained of her hand except bones and tendons and it was many months later before it was useful.

This was in the mid-twenties. It was typical of the numerous destructive and mutilating wound infections of that period, in the face of which doctors were helpless. Calvin Coolidge's son, Calvin Jr., was the victim of such an infection, caused by a blister on his heel acquired while playing tennis. This was a few years before the appearance of sulfanilamide, which probably would have saved him.

Erysipelas was another type of wound infection common in the decade of the twenties. It started in a small way from an abrasion or cut and spread outward in all directions, to be seen frequently on the face. It was lethal with new-born infants. The favored treatment was local applications of the messy black-syrupy compound ichthyol or magnesium sulphate compresses for as long as two to three weeks. We tried to check its spread by painting the spreading border with Lugol's Iodine (12% iodine) or freezing it with ethyl chloride spray. But nothing helped very much. Today it is very simple to treat with the sulfa drugs and some of the other antibiotics.

Scarlet fever, now so lightly regarded, was one of the very serious diseases we had to deal with because of the infections that could develop. There was the family of six children stricken one bitter February with a virulent type. My office nurse, the excellent Agnes McQuaig, volunteered to go to their small frame house and live with them for a month, through weather so cold at night that she put her fur coat on top of the bedding. Before it was over, two children had double running ears with one requiring a mastoid operation. Another child showed late severe kidney damage.

The advent of sulfa drugs in the mid-thirties would spell the abrupt end to such tissue infections as that of Annie's finger and erysipelas; and scarlet fever with its running ears and mastoid involvement would lose its terror. In the meantime, while all these marvels and others awaited us around the corner, general practitioners like myself in rural communities everywhere made do with what was available to us. By necessity, we could not treat our patients for specific complaints alone—we knew them and their problems too intimately. We had to see them whole.

IV. There Is No Such Thing As Unreal Pain

The emotions are strange and wonderful. My patients taught me many things, as I have said. Possibly most valuable of all, they showed me how to deal with feelings associated with the crises of life. How did they express grief? Certainly not as we see it so often on the stage, on television, and in novels—with loud weeping, wringing of hands and hysterics. In real life among my Anglo-Saxons, there was more sitting and standing about quietly with a stunned expression. They insisted on being in command of the situation, on making thoughtful suggestions, and on a minimum of fuss.

There comes to mind a mother who called me to her home one early evening. Her child of five had been accidentally killed by a blast from a shotgun held by a younger brother. Shotgun blasts mean strange-looking injuries and, in this case, it carried away half the child's neck without a drop of blood being visible anywhere. I found the mother quietly rocking with the dead child in her lap. She was weeping just a little and refused all sedatives and hypnotics. Her only words were, "I will be all right, please have the undertaker come at once."

On another occasion, a young man alone in a field was dynamiting large stones when an explosion occurred. By the time I arrived he was kneeling over a large rock, his face was bloody, he couldn't hear very well, one eye was closed and a hand was off at the wrist. He was just quietly swearing to himself. "Let's get to hospital," was the only thing he said.

When Sergeant McQuillin of the Metropolitan Toronto Police Force was slain by a bandit's bullet, I was asked to break the news to his mother who lived in the country. A tall handsome woman, she listened quietly, sat down and commented, "I hope he didn't suffer." She, also, refused all sedatives and hypnotics.

Individuals can recover from grief and wounds of the body but the worries and anxieties of life can cut very deep and affect every part of one's being.

As time went by I became more and more concerned about ill people themselves and relatively less about their illnesses. The patient gradually took precedence over his ailments. When I started medical practice, I was interested largely in the diseases and defects I might uncover; I was more disease-oriented than whole-person oriented. If I couldn't find such tell-tale evidence of ill health as fever, anemia, altered blood pressure, abnormal urine or just simple painful body spots, I felt I had failed my patient.

This shift in emphasis from disease to patient cannot be explained. I know that medicine itself was drifting that way, aiming more at treating people than diseases, but the shift in my interest did not come from the attitude of the profession. It came, perhaps, from the fact that I was seeing a lot of people who were ill but had no disease as disease was described in medical texts or had been demonstrated by my teachers, who were largely hospital instructors working among hospital patients. I am not particularly proud of this change in my primary concern as it may have resulted in a little less interest in keeping abreast of the technical aspects of medicine. We become most proficient in what we ponder and dream about, and I freely admit there were many family doctors of my era who knew more technical medicine than I did.

Yes, there were many people ill without any disease present. They came from many groups and the opportunities for helping them were endless. There were the young couples enthusiastically shouldering the burdens of married life who were confronted with problems stemming from sex, money, education, parents, etcetera. The middle-aged, too, had their problems planning the last half of their lives, and their difficulties so impressed me that I came to believe we needed guidance classes for this age group as urgently as for our teen-agers.

Young doctors of the 1920's and 1930's were ill-prepared to face the number of people we encountered with emotional difficulties. In medical schools psychiatry as we understand it today was practically unknown: it was for the birds! Psychiatric teaching was centered around the severely disturbed and the insane, and what general practitioners needed was psychiatry for the worried and anxious—what could be called "everyday psychiatry," to help their patients with the problems they had to live with day in and day out. The behavioral sciences were not yet offering to help us.

We were taught to think of the worst things first. We must never overlook an early cancer of the breast or cervix, and might succeed in detecting one every three years, whereas nearly every day some patient complained of a headache and the majority of these were tension headaches, on which little emphasis had been placed. We were left to improve our skills in handling emotional problems by observation and trial-and-error treatment.

Although we saw a lot of worried and anxious people, there were probably no more than at present. Estimates of their share of a family doctor's practice have varied from 10 to 60 per cent. The late Dr. A. G. McKerracher, Professor of Psychiatry at the University of Saskatchewan, probably came close to the truth when he suggested that 25 per cent of patients consulting Canadian general practitioners were doing so for reasons of anxiety and depression—with both sexes equally afflicted. Psychiatrists state that about 55 per cent of their patients are women and 45 per cent men.

About 25 per cent of my patients had purely emotional disorders or had an emotional overlay of physical ailments. This estimate applies over my thirty years of practice and not to any particular years. I say this because my competence in recognizing such disorders was not a constant skill. I had to learn as I went along, and so recognized more of them as I grew older.

Detection and identification called for unceasing curiosity about a patient's behavior, and my success depended upon how diligently I searched.

Really we know little in a medical way about anxiety, spleen, guilt, fear, remorse, etc. A doctor's business consists largely in finding out what puts these types of stress on people and what liberates them. We speak freely of "a healthy mind in a healthy body," as though these were distinct independent entities, which they certainly are not. But where in each individual does one begin and the other end? To ask the question another way: How do a person's emotions and physical body mesh?

A doctor regards a person as mentally ill or mentally unbalanced if his condition puts him into one of four distinct categories:

1. *Those suffering from neuroses*—people who, after a period of overwork, financial reverses, bereavement or insomnia become tense, on-edge, irritable, worried and anxious—and then perhaps feel some discomfort in their head, stomach, chest, or abdomen. Such a person may still have steady nerves, be cool, collected, well-adjusted and intelligent, and after a rest or vacation, a few nights' good sleep, and perhaps the taking of a sedative, will become less irritable and anxious. An anxiety is a mild neurosis; a depression is a more serious neurosis. As a rule, the neuroses do not lead to a serious break with the realities of life.

2. *Those who suffer from psychoses* are subject to severe mental and often behavior disorders, resulting frequently in a break with reality. A person with a psychosis, in the words of some of my Scottish patients, was said to have "gone wrong." More generally, they are described as insane, crazy or mad.

Like the neurotic, the psychotic has a mental conflict, but it is more severe, so severe that he seems to be living in another world. He might be seeing something that doesn't exist, hearing voices where there are none and doing inappropriate things to himself and to others. His judgment may be so impaired that a court of law might commit him to a mental hospital, although there is no definition of insanity that will stand up in a court of law.

There is a small group of persons who hear fancied voices or see things not there, who are not necessarily psychotic or even neurotic. Like Moses, or Paul of Tarsus, or Joan of Arc, or perhaps Saint Patrick, they can be very intense people dedicated to ideas.

3. *Abnormal personalities*—best described as hysterical people.

4. *Mentally retarded and mentally sub-normal.*

The neuroses are the least serious of mental disorders and the most common. I agree with a psychologist who said, "Every person is entitled to one neurosis or mental breakdown in the course of a lifetime." However, the emotional conflict in a neurosis is a serious disruption to a patient's well-being, because for the time being it is dominating his personality.

By amateurish ways I had to learn how to understand the worried and anxious and how to feel at home in this field. Little help came from my teachers or textbooks, and the knowledge I gained through experiences from which the following are taken may seem simple and obvious to doctors today.

Albert, nineteen years old, called at two o'clock one winter's night from his home some five miles distant. Alone in the house in an upstairs bedroom, he informed me that he wanted to be emasculated. He had a large wicked-looking instrument used to crush the testicles of animals which he had tried on himself but had found too painful. The skin of his scrotum was bruised, so I had to believe that he had attempted to mutilate himself. There had been some trouble with a girl and he didn't want anything more to do with sex. He gave no further details and I didn't ask.

I suggested that sexual sterilization might not be the answer to his problem. "You aren't the first to react this way. This feeling will pass and you may want to get married in a few years and have a family. Don't make a hasty move—think it over. Put that instrument back in the barn where it belongs and come in and see me in a few days."

He returned in a week to thank me for the advice, adding, "I am planning marriage and everything is grand."

Ethel, a bright young mother with an infant child, consulted me because she was worried over family affairs, including an ill husband who disliked his occupation of farming. With little income, she didn't know where to turn. Her chief concern seemed to be how to advise her husband about employment and his vocation. How much pressure should she bring to bear on him to do what she wanted? I didn't know the half of her difficulties, but I stood in some awe of the depth of her insight. The best I could do was to listen sympathetically. Two years later, when the family had moved to another locality, I received a letter from Ethel which is one of my prized possessions. It read in part:

> "I still remember with nostalgia the 'good medicine' you dispensed—not always by pill or noxious liquid. I shall never forget the time I thought I needed psychiatry—to your amusement. Little you knew—I never did tell all. You let me talk my head off and talked back a bit too. Then you shook your head and with real regret in your voice said, 'I haven't helped a bit.' That sentence and the voice it was said in was just the help that took me over the hump. I don't know why, but that was the most cheering thing ever said to my despair."

These patients, Albert and Ethel, taught me several important things which were later confirmed by other worried folk. In discussing patients' emotional problems, I must never tell them what to do; I must let them make the decisions. I must not moralize or sit in judgment as this would be irrelevant and often unmerciful. It was not my business to assign guilt or innocence. Secondly, it was not necessary to probe deeply into the details of their emotional conflicts in order to bring a lot of relief. I had an inborn conviction about this as it has always seemed to me unwholesome to wallow in one's indiscretions, difficulties and mistakes—as the psychoanalyst invites one to do.

Dwelling on my own mistakes was unhealthy for me and has led me to believe it is better to forget errors as quickly as possible and just vow not to repeat them.

This was in marked contrast to what the psychoanalysts were telling us in the early thirties. Their treatment took the form of interviews with the patient reclining on a couch and the standard program of treatment was one hour five days a week, eleven months a year for three years at a cost of five dollars per interview. I respected the psychoanalysts highly because they were the most intensively trained specialists around. In addition to a long post-graduate internship, they were required to psychoanalyze patients under supervision and be psychoanalyzed themselves. But it was discouraging for a family doctor to gather from psychoanalytic procedures useful ideas he could adopt for the better treatment of the worried and mentally disturbed. Fortunately, many psychoanalysts have now abandoned their long programs of therapy and are using shorter and sharper interviews with patients and whole families. They report this is easier and more realistic psychiatry.

Leslie, twenty-two years of age, complained of stomach distress in the early morning and before lunch. Considerable questioning revealed that his wife, whom I was not attending, was several months pregnant, and his symptoms were precisely those of morning sickness. From the experience of a friend, he had been led to expect to react like his wife. The symptoms disappeared in a few days. On telling my wife of this curious case, she skeptically remarked, "It must be very unusual for a husband to be so concerned." It is rare; I had read about it but wasn't sure this sympathetic type of dyspepsia occurred until I met this young man.

A country girl of five years was getting unpredictable attacks of asthma—not severe but troublesome. She was robust, the eldest of three children. I couldn't even suggest a cause. The mother solved the problem of diagnosis. The girl was a bit of a tomboy and loved to go to the barn to help her father. When this was refused, she had an attack. On settling to the girl's satisfaction how often and when she could go to the barn, the asthma disappeared.

Psychiatry is the most recently born baby of medical science which deals with the relationship of mind and body and it really represents a return of medicine to its more humane and personal beginnings. Every new science has growing pains and one of psychiatry's difficulties has been simplifying its findings to easily understood terms. A personal incident was an early landmark for me.

During my early twenties I smoked cigarettes fairly heavily except during several fitful attempts to stop. On these occasions I found it comforting to chew the stem of a match. I know this was not a rational action and it may slightly indicate the type of person I am. While chewing on a match during one of the periods of abstinence I coughed violently. On inhaling, down went the match and stuck in my throat. It was nine in the morning. My throat became sorer and sorer and by noon I concluded that it would be a sensible action to see a doctor. It was a warm day in June and I was in my shirt sleeves. As I was going out of the office door to consult my confrère down the street, I spied the match in my shirt pocket; it wasn't in my throat at all. I turned back to talk to myself, because it appeared I couldn't trust my throat to tell me whether or not it harbored a match. Apparently, the match had dropped into my throat, scratched it slightly and popped out again. My throat felt fine in a few minutes. Assuredly it appeared that I was a neurotic of some type.

Whether this was true or not, the experience helped explain why I often had so much trouble convincing people there was no fishbone in their throats when they were sure there was. Some patients were positive they could feel the bone, even after I had removed one, and there was certainly nothing in the throat. My routine procedure was to examine the throat carefully, remove the bone if one was present, then paint the throat with an analgesic solution, give a Luminal tablet and a couple of aspirins and ask the patient to go home for a few hours. If his throat still bothered him at the end of that time would he please return and let me have another look. They were all sure they would be back, but few returned.

How could I explain what was happening to them? I learned

I must never use the words *imagine* or *imagination*. I must never tell them they imagined there was a fishbone in their throat; it would be insulting. Nor could I tell a patient with a headache or pain that he imagined it. *There is no such thing as an unreal pain or headache.* Patients are nearly always correct about their symptoms, but may be very wrong as to the cause. If a patient has a pain and we find nothing, it is our failure. If we give the impression that it is all in his mind, he will be annoyed and will probably go elsewhere.

The alternative to using the word "imagination" is to tell the patient that he is hypersensitive to pain, has a low threshold to pain, or that his subconscious mind is playing tricks on him. Most people will accept the last explanation and this was my favorite.

There is another way of looking at my little episode, when I was erroneously sure there was a match in my throat. Each body organ has a means of telling us when something ails it. It may be by pain, tremor, overactivity as when the bowels develop diarrhaea, or coughing from lung infection. Each organ may be considered to have its own language of distress.

My second landmark in gaining insight into the mechanics of emotions was supplied by a patient. It was a clear instance of a body organ expressing itself.

William was a middle-aged, successful business man. He complained so often of being ill when I found little wrong that I despaired of ever understanding him. On a couple of occasions I felt like asking him to consult another doctor. This went on for several years, until one night he presented me with a clue to at least some of his illnesses.

It was one o'clock at night in his home and I was listening to him complain that he had appendicitis. As he lay naked on the bed a remarkable thing happened. A strip of muscle about one and a half inches wide on his lower right chest wall, which extended around to the mid-line of the upper right abdomen, began slowly twitching rhythmically. With each spasm he cried out. To the non-medical person this might seem to be a natural and frequent occurrence. It is not. The only experience I had had with anything similar was an occasional rhythmic twitching of my own upper eyelid, lasting only a few minutes. I had never heard of large muscles like those of the chest wall being thrown into rhythmic spasm, nor had I ever read of the like. William's muscle spasm had a far-reaching effect on him. When the muscle spasm occurred where he considered an appendix pain would be, it followed that it must mean appendicitis. At this point his subconscious mind took over and gave him some true symptoms of appendicitis, including nausea. He was sick to his stomach when he called me.

To follow this a little further, one of William's frequent complaints was kidney trouble with pain in one flank. The pain gave him other symptoms he thought should go with kidney trouble, namely, frequent urination with some burning sensation. It now seemed possible that internal muscles in his flank were contracting when he had this kidney pain.

Before I was William's physician, he had had a prolonged spell of severe and intractable headaches. Examination in a city hospital by a consultant with all the tests he could think of, including electro-encephalography and the painful injection of air into the brain ventricles, revealed nothing to explain the headaches. Now in the light of my new knowledge it seemed reasonable to suppose that the headaches were due to a spasm of some of the arteries of his brain. I say this because psychiatrists now teach that involuntary muscles such as those of the bowel and blood vessels can go into spasm just as the voluntary muscles of our limbs and trunk do.

William showed me a whole new dimension to our feelings. He was contending with a major imbalance between his nervous system and the rest of his body. There may be many people with various degrees of such an imbalance. It suggests how far our feelings can lead us astray as to their cause.

One of the first things I learned from worried and anxious people was to listen long and carefully to what they had to say and to allow time for thoughtful answers to my questions. This is really time-consuming because most of us don't know what we believe about many things until we have said it. I must never be in a hurry; I must not even look at my watch during an interview. A watch out of sight below my desk on the floor would have been helpful but I never did put one there.

I should in all fairness add that the physician interested in emotional problems soon learns with surprise and relief that repeated sessions of psychotherapy may be no more time-consuming than repeated physical examinations. And there is another reward: many of the neurotic and unstable people who came to me, even the so-called sinful and wayward ones, proved to be among the most interesting individuals I ever met. Not knowing them would have been my loss.

We are all at times depressed, anxious, irritable, tense, and suffer an inferiority complex. In fact, the most successful of us are apt to worry the most. As I worked with these patients, it seemed very important not to forget that hope is as important in relieving emotional conflicts as anxiety is in causing them.

In my search over the years for hidden emotional problems I came upon people in odd and revealing predicaments. One person I cannot forget was Minnie, who was a veritable storehouse of strange conflicts. When she first consulted me she was twenty-seven years old, an attractive woman, smartly dressed, with two fine boys. She complained of "choking" and strangling spells which lasted until her face became a dark color, and explained that they went back in time to an operation she had had six months earlier. She admitted to being a nervous person, saying that stress and excitement did occasionally bring on the attacks, but she was sure that in general her nervousness had nothing to do with causing them.

We were both standing in my office, I behind her as I examined her ears with a speculum, when I gave her a minor fright by stamping hard on the floor. Promptly she had a "choking" spell. It was a spasm of the larynx with a crowing inspiration and lasted until she was quite distressed. Her ailment was obviously nervous in origin and called for a careful examination and a complete history. And what a history she gave me!

She told me that at nine months of age she had had a septic

sore throat followed by "leakage of the heart" resulting in convulsive seizures throughout childhood. These seizures had persisted to the present time but without her body stiffening. They came on without provocation and, I presumed, were epileptic in nature, of the mild type.

Six months before I saw her, in a car accident she suffered a skull fracture, two broken legs, and a broken arm. And the previous year her uterus had been removed. Now to all these troubles were added some marital difficulties. I had no way of checking on the truthfulness of the statements about her past history as she had lived in many different places, but it was obvious that her nervous system had taken quite a battering.

As for her "choking" spells, I explained that these were nervous in origin, that she was in no real danger, that she had been under such stress her subconscious mind was playing tricks with her; that people cannot divest themselves easily of overacting emotions, that it is not like turning the knob on the radio, but more like a musician learning a new score—and, finally, that we really cannot help a distressed person who doesn't want to get well. It was not very effective therapy as it acted slowly. However, in two months' time she was having fewer and milder choking spells.

Unfortunately, by this time she was coming in frequently with a variety of fresh complaints. On one occasion it was fainting and dizzy spells, another time it was insomnia, and several times just plain weariness. When she came to report that she was having vaginal bleeding I was really stumped as this was a woman who had had her uterus removed.

Still this was not all. In time a new and unexpected complaint appeared. She was developing numerous hemorrhages under the skin called purpuric spots. They were one-half to one inch across and painful. They first appeared on her face and arms and later on her legs and back. Over a period of several months I saw more than a hundred of them come and go. On one occasion I counted nineteen on her thighs and six on her back, the latter group indicating to me that the purpuric spots were not self-inflicted by bruising or otherwise injuring herself.

During this time she was carefully examined during two prolonged periods in a city hospital. Many hundreds of dollars were spent on the investigations, to say nothing of doctors' time. The only conclusion possible seemed to be that the purpuric spots were further evidence of what her feelings and emotions were doing to her before any full-fledged nervous breakdown occurred. She was a casualty in more ways than one to the severe stresses of life.

Today's psychiatrists probably would classify Minnie as a hysterical personality, not a neurotic. Hysteria is one of the grossly abnormal manifestations of personality and in itself is not a dangerous ailment. But it is so puzzling it is of particular interest. With hysteria we never find out how much is due to conscious processes and how much is due to unconscious processes. Under no circumstances can we ever put ourselves 100 per cent into another person's shoes: there is always a credibility gap. With hysteria, the gap is very great indeed.

I mentioned Minnie's vaginal bleeding in the absence of a uterus. She still had a vagina from which the bleeding could come. The saints of old, according to secular and religious history, often developed bleeding from various sources—nose bleeds, vaginal hemorrhages and even blood dripping from the fingers.

Minnie's was an extreme case. Two other histories dealt with more run-of-the-mill emotional problems.

A prosperous intelligent farmer of fifty-five suddenly became listless, tired, unable to sleep, avoided company, and was indifferent to the conduct of his business. He offered no clue or explanation for his condition. On my reminding him that he had consulted me years earlier, he admitted he felt then as he did now.

On the earlier occasion, though it was not mentioned, we both knew that his mother had just died in a mental hospital and a sister had recently been discharged from one. A physical examination had proved normal and I concluded that his chief difficulty was worry about his own health. He was given small doses of Luminal and told to work hard because mixing a liberal amount of muscle activity with nervous tension is wholesome therapy. In three weeks he was well again and very grateful. He had remained in good health until the present consultation.

This time a different fear was operating. For a cancer of the cheek, which was now healed for several months, he had received radium therapy. He thought it possible but couldn't agree, that there might be subconscious concern about this cheek lesion. He was quite sure he was prepared for anything. Nevertheless, he was willing to cooperate and, given the same therapy as before, he reacted with the same happy results.

Somewhat similar was the history of James, a successful hard-working carpenter-farmer. For six months he had felt a lump in his throat and was sure it was cancer. Though it became more troublesome a few days after the burial of his brother, he was satisfied that this event had nothing to do with his throat discomfort as he had known for some time that his brother was dying. His throat was particularly bad in the mornings when he must thoroughly chew every bite of meat or he would choke.

A difficulty we had had with this patient five years earlier came to mind and I looked up his file. At that time it had taken two months of effort by examination, consultation, and reassurances to convince him his lungs were healthy. The key to his difficulty then was the death of a brother in childhood from tuberculosis; my patient, who suffered from chronic nasal catarrh, was sure that some day it would turn into tuberculosis and lay him low.

As on the earlier occasion, I explained in a rather ineffectual manner that there was nothing seriously wrong, nothing more than his subconscious mind taking over temporarily. However, I granted that I must prove to him the reasonableness of my diagnosis; if I wasn't doing this to his satisfaction, I begged him to return and give me another chance. After a couple of months, with much effort on his part and after enlisting the aid of his wife, he was able to convince himself there was no lump in his throat.

It can be argued that my friend Walter T. does not belong in a discussion of illness due to emotional disturbance. But perhaps he does, as an opposite example of a healthy mind in a healthy body. If he was concerned about the disabilities attending the ageing process, he brought humor and common sense to bear upon his difficulties, and in doing so he taught me a lesson I shall always remember on the resiliency of the human spirit.

Walter T. was for many years a Methodist minister in our community, until forced to leave his profession when his voice failed him. Then he devoted himself to managing a hundred-barrel-a-day flour mill he had inherited. He was a little man of 5′4″ and like many small men he compensated for his short stature by finding enough energy to present a forceful posture and a dynamic presence at all times. He needed every bit of ability and energy he could muster as the small flour mills were steadily being squeezed out by the giants like the Lake of the Woods Mill. Long before I became his physician, Walter had the habit of dropping into my office to discuss most anything that struck his fancy, or to show me a new book. He was a great reader. His visits were a welcome diversion for he was alert and entertaining. Even in his later years he had a photographic memory and, given an unfamiliar page to read, would immediately repeat it back—maybe not word for word, but at least 80 per cent correct.

A phone call came in one busy Saturday afternoon: "Walter speaking. Come and see me."

"What is the matter?"

"This is my seventieth birthday."

"But Walter," I protested, "my waiting room is full. I will be there in a couple of hours."

"That isn't good enough. I must see you now."

"Very well," I agreed. I had learned from experience not to say no to his imperious commands, so I announced to the patients waiting that I had an emergency and would be back shortly. I had only a block to travel.

Walter met me in his living room surrounded by his children. "Doctor, what did they do for King David on his seventieth birthday?" he demanded.

"Walter, I haven't the slightest idea."

"Here is a Bible. Please read to me the first four verses of Chapter I, The First Book of Kings."

I did as I was told:

"Now King David was old and stricken in years; and they covered him with clothes, but he gat no heat.

"Wherefore his servants said unto him, 'Let there be sought for my Lord the king a young virgin: and let her stand before the king, and let her cherish him; and let her lie in thy bosom, that my lord the king may get heat.'

"So they sought for a fair damsel throughout all the coasts of Israel, and found Abishag a Shunammite, and brought her to the king.

"And the damsel was very fair and she cherished the king and ministered to him; but the king knew her not."

When I had finished reading Walter rose and confronted me.

"You have read what they did for King David on his seventieth birthday. My family have given me an electric blanket. Do you think we have made much progress?"

My day was made and I returned to my full waiting room with zest.

Depression is a warning signal I learned to heed. I saw only a dozen or so suicides in my practice, but these plus the many people with depressive illness who were potential suicides added up to a significant problem.

The main street of Lucknow is Ontario Highway No. 86. On its east-west course ten miles west of the village this highway goes through the center of a cemetery of the Scots community of Lochalsh. Why this highway through a cemetery? It was started in the 1830's on the south side of the road. Some years later a native son hanged himself. The local citizens with their Calvinist leanings were particular about who was in their burial ground. He was laid to rest alone on the north side of the road. Since then so many of his neighbors have followed him there that the road now seems to divide the cemetery into equal parts.

Most of the elder citizens of my area disapproved of suicide, probably for one or more of the following reasons: It seemed

1) a sin against our Maker, or 2) a cowardly way of settling a problem, or 3) ungentlemanly and even bad manners to embarrass the relatives this way.

When I started practice I felt that death by suicide was a disgraceful act and surely must be the product of a seriously unbalanced mind. This belief did not stem from my medical school training, where we were given little information about suicides beyond the warning that depressed people were likely to resort to it. Nor were my opinions a reflection of my Methodist upbringing. The suicides themselves changed my thinking about them as through the years they persuaded me that a sane person can do away with himself and that self-destruction can be a reasoned act.

How did they teach me? In the first place, they weren't long in appearing.

Ethel consulted me during my first year of practice. She was a plumply beautiful dark-haired vivacious girl of about twenty. It was Easter and she talked about her first year in university, which was about to end. She was afraid she might fail the term examinations and her parents were most concerned that their only child succeed. The situation was complicated a little, but not much, by a torrid love affair with a man of a different religious faith. I couldn't decide why she came to me or even whether she wanted advice. It seemed she just wanted to talk. She was not from my village and I knew her only in a casual way.

The day following her visit she drove alone to the family's Muskoka cottage and drowned by jumping into the cold April lake. For me this was acutely disturbing. I had failed completely in assessing one of my first depressed patients.

As stated, Ethel was a university student. Almost every spring one or two high school students would interview me voluntarily or by direction of their parents. Their story was always the same: they were discouraged about their examinations, couldn't sleep and often couldn't eat. They all feared a "nervous breakdown."

Why do high school and university students crack up?

Stengel* points out that suicide rates in England among university students are higher than in corresponding age groups of the general population. In Oxford and Cambridge they are five to six times in excess of expectation and lower but still excessive in a group of provincial universities.

At a recent Canadian Medical Association annual convention Dr. D. L. McNeil of Calgary advised that "virtually all university students who kill themselves are male." Backing this up was Dr. G. E. Wodehouse of Toronto, who has studied the subject for fifteen years and who thinks most students judge themselves and life too rigidly.

The most enlightening comments on this have come to me from a man who has become a very successful professional inventor after spending two years in my village twenty years ago. He was unable to pass his second-year high school examination and insists that if he had finished high school he could not have become an inventor because nowhere else but out in the harsh world could he learn to trust only what he could prove. Of course, his accomplishments as an inventor don't necessarily make him an authority on one of the problems arising out of the boom in higher education, but he seems to speak rationally when he says, "There is too much pressure on students to get high marks. Rather, we should teach them humility—if their marks are high, to appreciate that this is only a beginning and, if low, that it is no disaster; it is instead an indication they should try something else and continue searching until they find something they like." We tend to expect our young people to choose a vocation too hurriedly. How can they know whether or not they will like certain fields of activity until they try them? And this takes time. If a person is to fulfill himself it is paramount that he find a vocation he likes whether it is selling cars in a car lot, shirts over a counter, or building a spiral stairway.

* Erwin Stengel, *Suicide and Attempted Suicide*. Great Britain, Penguin Books, Ltd., 1964.

(Doctors are poor examplars in this matter. Referring to obituaries and causes of death reported in the *Journal of the American Medical Association*, Dr. Singer told the Third International Congress of Social Psychiatry that U.S. psychiatrists averaged 58 suicides per 100,000 population between May 1965 and May 1969. This is almost 300 per cent higher than the country's national population average of 15 per 100,000. Additional data he presented showed that the average per 100,000 for other specialties was: anesthesiologists 44, urologists and G.P.s 34 each. American surgeons were ninth on the list with an average of 22 suicides per 100,000, followed by pediatricians and radiologists with 17 per 100,000, which is close to the national average.)

Students despair too soon, but the will to give up can present itself at any age.

Mrs. C. and her husband lived together for fifty years in reasonable harmony, until Mr. C. died after a short bout with pneumonia when nearly eighty. On the day before his burial, she went to bed declaring, "I am going to die with Calvin. I cannot live without him." She was a thin little creature and as she flitted about her small frame house in her black nun's veiling it seemed that a slight breeze could carry her away. Although frail, she had a will of iron. She had decided to die, she carried it through and was buried within ten days of the demise of her husband—leaving her house in perfect order, clean as a pin. As her mind was bright and keen to the last and I couldn't find anything physically wrong except her age which was eighty plus, I had to conclude that she was sane.

We read of people in darkest Africa under the influence of witch doctors deciding to die. Mrs. C. was the only person I saw in my years of practice who voluntarily chose death and speedily accomplished it without a violent act. I can't say that I tried very hard to dissuade her. I advised, "Just think it over carefully again."

I have a deep respect for the convictions of elderly people about living on. They have experienced most of what life has to offer and know much more clearly what continuing life means to them individually than I could ever guess. When a person never again has a worthwhile task to perform, when his day is spent looking at the ceiling, why hold him back?

Perhaps there was one other person who quietly and with dignity determined his own ending. Adam, a robust farmer of seventy, went to bed because of stomach ulcers and stoutly refused all food and medication. Whenever I raised the question of food he turned his face to the wall and would not discuss it. He drank some water at intervals but resolutely stuck to his decision about food and accomplished his end in six weeks. I tried quite hard to change his thinking. I classified him as a sick person because he showed evidences of senile mind changes.

It is true that when we speak of suicides we usually mean those who destroy themselves by violent means. Many, by this reasoning, would not classify Mrs. C. and Adam as suicides; they would prefer to think of them as meeting in an unusual way the problems of old age and the declining years.

The man who was our family physician for many years shot himself. An autopsy showed him in the final stages of abdominal cancer. To me his suicide had more elements of courage than cowardice, though it was difficult to forgive him for not telling his family and neglecting to leave at least a note. But had I been in his shoes, what final message could I have given that would be heartening to anyone? He was a sick man and none of us knows what we will think or feel when we are fatally stricken. We may think we know, but a seriously ill person is as different from a well person as a sheep is different when isolated from the flock.

Someone has said, "When a man pronounces himself a prisoner, there are two courses open before him, one of which he must take. He must burst aside the bars of his prison house, or he must in one way or another commit suicide." Our family doctor's self-inflicted end was not a despicable action.

A. E. Hotchner reports that Ernest Hemingway discussed his approaching suicide in these words: "If I can't exist on my own terms, then existence is impossible, do you understand? That is how I have lived, and that is how I must live—or not live." Hotchner comments that Hemingway, a man of writing prowess, did not wish to live without that prowess. Its loss was one of the forces that crushed him.

Down through the ages, the cause of suicides has baffled the leaders of civilization and the medical profession. There has been a wide range of thinking on the subject. In ancient Greece and Rome attitudes varied from condemnation to admiration. Sigerist writes: "In Greek society there was a stigma attached to the sick man. To be sure, it was not the stigma of sinfulness but rather the stigma of being less worthy or inferior. The Stoics sought to go beyond the classic position in that they looked upon health and sickness as the two sides of the same coin, with vice the only genuine evil and virtue the one genuine good." An incurable disease was held to be sufficient reason for suicide. Some philosophers of all ages have recommended suicide as the perfect way of gaining freedom from suffering. Zeno, a philosopher of the fifth century B.C., hanged himself because of a broken finger. Nietzsche, the German philosopher of the nineteenth century, wrote, "The thought of suicide is a great comfort and helps one over many a bad night."

A bank manager in mid-life suffered what is called a sub-arachnoid hemorrhage. This is a brain hemorrhage, but not the type causing a stroke. With good nursing care available, he was treated at home. He was dangerously ill, slowly recovered and resumed his bank duties six months later. But his illness left him with a changed personality. Nearly everything bothered him unduly. The officials of the bank were informed of this but chose to take no action. Then one day a bank inspector questioned a loan he had approved as manager. That evening he ended it all by drinking two ounces of Lysol. Why do people choose such agonizing and unimaginative means of destruction? The urge to do so must be most compulsive. I failed this man and his family badly; he should have been watched more carefully. He was sick and I didn't even suspect he might turn to suicide so readily when provoked.

A recent widower of about 65 consulted me; he was very lonely without his wife. He had been an outstanding success in business and farming. I admired him and was proud to consider myself one of his friends. He wanted my help because he was depressed, couldn't sleep, and was losing weight. On questioning him, he spoke freely of the urge he had at times to end his life. In particular, he was frightened of heights. He found the urge to suicide could come on suddenly, at unexpected times, with almost irresistible force. I gave him Luminal tablets and talked to him. He returned in a week, grateful for his improvement and ready to pay me several times my fee. This type of interview was repeated on several occasions during the following six months—until one morning I was called to a fire in one of his houses in which he had burned to death.

After looking the situation over, I discussed the matter with his two sons.

"Do you see what I see? Your father let the cat and dog out and was lying just inside the main entrance with the door locked and the keys on a nearby table. It looks like a possible suicide."

"Yes," they assured me, "we agree that's what probably happened. We knew about his depressed feelings and his calls on you."

"Did he make his will?"

"Yes, everything is in order."

"I must call the coroner," I advised them. "He is an elderly man and lives thirty miles from here. Shall I tell him this is a suicide?"

"Please do not."

I obeyed their wishes. The coroner didn't appear to suspect the truth and I thereby may have contributed to the unreliable Canadian statistics on suicides.

Later I discussed my action on this occasion with a senior coroner who suggested that the elderly coroner possibly didn't tell all he saw; that coroners learn from experience not to sign a death certificate as a suicide unless they can prove it. Lacking proof, the sensible decision is to call it an accidental death. He cited a death where a man parked his car close to a railway track and while repairing a tire was struck and killed by a passing train. The inquest jury brought in a verdict of accidental death, though the foreman later confided that they believed it was a suicide because the victim knew the train schedules, was known to be depressed, and examination of the car tires showed there was nothing wrong with them. They just couldn't prove it was suicide, so why say so? Possibly there should be another category of suspected or possible suicides.

Tom in his early years had his private bank. This was followed by a period of twenty-five years or so when he derived an income from loans to farmers and tradesmen. He charged 12% interest—6% for himself and 6% for the bank from which he said he obtained the money. The local public generally regarded this as very excessive interest and thought of Tom as a hard man, a usurer.

This was scarcely a just judgment as the loans served a very useful purpose. With them he gave many a man a start in life who couldn't have secured financial means anywhere else. Also, his interest rate could hardly qualify him today as a usurer.

At age sixty-five the harsh judgment of the public got through to Tom. He was a sensitive soul. The Christmas before his death he confided to me that a farmer had brought him the gift of a chicken, adding the pathetic confession, "I didn't know anyone thought enough of me for that." With his heightened sensitivity he became morbidly concerned about illnesses of his acquaintances. He was wont to accost me on the street with, "How is my sick friend so-and-so? What ails him?" This in spite of the fact that my answer always was, "I am not at liberty to say."

One early winter morning he walked out into the icy waters of Lake Huron and lay down. I didn't think of Tom as a potential suicide. I was not his physician, but if I had been I would have known of no way to change his feeling of hopelessness.

These last two patients illustrate the difficulty I had in identifying people so gloomy they were likely to commit suicide.

How could I know whether the man saddened by the death of his wife, and Tom, hurt that his neighbors shunned him, would recover spontaneously or not from their melancholy or give way to it by self-destruction? Depression of spirits is one of the most common maladies of man and one of the most varied. One man's annoying melancholy may be another man's despair. For years doctors have been cautioned to expect suicide by depressed people. But how depressed must they be? There are no recognized degrees of severity of depression by which to establish a rational classification that would distinguish a temporary mood of pessimism from a covert but firm desire to die.

While we await a workable classification of depressions based on their severity, probably it is wisest to consider that all obviously depressed folk are prone to suicide just as those are who are low to a morbid degree. In any case a threat of suicide is a serious warning.

From my limited experience I conclude that suicidal urges do not seem to spring from environment but rather to be built into the individual.

Depressions are serious neuroses. The endogenous depression, that is a depression proceeding from within, is as near to being a clinical entity as almost any disease in medicine. Its treatment is no longer a sacred preserve of the psychiatrist. It is part of general medicine and certainly part of family medicine where the condition is quite common.

The teachings of religion in regard to suicide are interesting and are thought to sway many. But religious taboos do not necessarily dictate a nation's suicide rate.

Islam condemns suicide unconditionally. While neither the Old nor the New Testament forbids suicide explicitly, the Koran does so in several instances. It even declares suicide to be a much greater crime than homicide. The Old Testament mentions only four cases of suicide, the best known being those of Samson and King Saul, both of whom killed themselves to avoid death by the enemy. The Christian church of the Middle Ages condemned suicide as a form of murder and at one period ordained that the body of the suicide be refused a Christian burial.

Granting that statistics are notably suspect for many countries, some generalizations are interesting. The Catholic Republic of Ireland and Catholic Italy are said to have quite low suicide rates, whereas Catholic Austria has one of the highest in the world. The welfare state does not markedly effect the situation, as witness Denmark and Sweden who are far above the world average, while Norway and Great Britain are well below it. In Egypt, a Moslem country where suicide is judged a disgrace, the low official figure given is not to be trusted.

As for the complexities of today's living, so often blamed for so much, they do not account for some of the high suicide rates. In the United States, for instance, where deaths by suicide are relatively high, higher than in Canada, the statistics for 1900 and 1959 varied hardly at all, though there had been a perceptible decline during the two world wars. Why?

I cannot leave the subject of suicide having given the impression that all was darkness and frustration for me in this realm of practice. In 1933, at the bottom of the depression, a patient frequently came in to see me, just wanting to talk; he might appear any time of the day. He was one of twelve directors of a large optics firm in Cleveland, with relatives in our village. It worried and depressed him that his colleagues were keeping the factory open at a loss to give employees part-time work; he didn't see how they could continue the policy much longer. Three directors had already destroyed themselves and he was fearful for himself. That he weathered the storm safely may have been due in small part to the help I gave him.

Possibly I helped others. Failures are easy to identify and assess. But how can you take credit for those who recover when they might have done so unaided?

V. The Strangest of All Man's Maladies

Addictions to alcohol and other drugs are now considered illnesses involving the emotions. Many doctors believe they are the strangest of all man's maladies.

In the 1920's I was seeing three or four narcotic addicts each year; they were morphine users and they were transients. I mean by this that they came into town by train one day and left the next. While there, they would make the rounds of the doctors' offices and sometimes the dentists'. On one occasion a desperate man went through the transom of a dentist's office to steal the drug.

I saw only one local morphine addict. Irwin (this was not his real name) came to the village as a businessman when he was elderly and already an addict. Few knew of his addiction, however, when two years later he shot himself through the heart with a .22 by pulling the trigger with his toe. I don't know how long he had been addicted, but it was long enough to break up his family and to prove after three tries that he could never again build a profitable business. Yet he was alert, bright, and sane when he destroyed himself, though he was a sick man.

It is interesting that all the transient morphine addicts were young men. Each was in great misery from sweating and shaking as he pleaded for a small hypo of morphine. Largely out of sympathy, I always granted the request though I was convinced that it was illegal to do so. However, from a recent review of the federal narcotic legislation of that period, I learn that I was in error about any culpability.

In the early twenties narcotic addiction was understood to

include addiction to morphine, heroin and opium. The Narcotic Control Act, administered by the Narcotic Division of the Department of Health, Ottawa, was aimed particularly at wiping out opium smoking among the Chinese of Vancouver. Doctors were required to keep a record of their narcotic purchases and be prepared to submit such records at any time to the Department of Health. They could use the drugs for medicinal purposes such as treatment of cancer, but the regulations did not precisely spell out the full scope of a doctor's responsibility, and no mention whatever was made of hypodermics to occasional patients. The laws indicated concern about doctors who were very free with their prescriptions and also about doctors who were themselves narcotic users. In 1928 a young doctor in Toronto was convicted of prescribing narcotics for self-administration and was given a three-month jail sentence. Apparently the authorities placed more emphasis on punitive measures than on treatment.

Then in the early thirties the transient addicts stopped coming and I saw no more of them. I believe a considerable number were now being treated in jails. Also there were fewer in the country as a whole. Statistics for 1923 show 9000 narcotic addicts in Canada; with this number decreasing to 4000 in the early thirties. The decrease can be explained in part by the fact that after 1925 regulations of the Narcotic Control Act were tightened and in 1927 it became necessary for a prescription to be in the doctor's handwriting; pharmacists could not honor telephone requests. The RCMP started using undercover agents posing as addicts to interview doctors and ask for narcotics. Some spotters were former addicts.

Because alcoholism was not regarded as an illness, the personal reasons for people's abuse of alcohol did not come under a doctor's purview. A drunk was a drunk, and if he became offensive the local police took him in charge. It was as simple as that. Although doctors were thought to be authorities on living wholesome and satisfying lives, they were in fact only authorities on the treatment of diseases and injuries—which is something quite different. Or to repeat what was said before, my medical training, as that of my confrères, was disease-and-injury oriented and not whole-person oriented. As my interests and attitudes changed with the passing years and my experience broadened, I learned from the alcoholics I encountered a great deal about hidden stresses, their effects and alleviation.

Mr. B. had been a so-called dried-out alcoholic for three years. He hadn't taken a drink during that time, but always had a supply of liquor on hand. He was an absorbingly interesting conversationalist, but never talked about his drinking problem. On several social occasions his wife seized some opportunity to announce, "It's like walking on an icy sidewalk waiting for the time when Jim will take his first drink." She seemed to miss the old difficult days and almost to be anticipating his fall. She was typical of the many spouses who are of little help in handling their alcoholic partners and are, in fact, a deterrent to treatment.

A successful business man, with his kind understanding nature and never-failing cheerfulness was one of the most popular men in the community. In mid-life he became a thorough-going alcoholic and, on the pleading of his wife and her brother, I persuaded him while still drinking to go to Toronto and spend a couple of weeks in the Dr. Gordon Bell Alcoholism Clinic. Two days later Dr. Bell telephoned to report that our patient was sober and wished to go home. Of course I agreed, as he was a voluntary patient. Not long afterwards, on the main street in the village, he gave me a proper calling down. "All the people down there are failures in business and cannot stop drinking. I want you to understand I am neither of those. Doctor, don't ever do that to me again."

Denial is a characteristic of the alcoholic. Our businessman never admitted to uncontrolled drinking and I was his physician until his death at seventy years from pneumonia. Of course, he was an alcoholic. He was drinking daily and frequently to excess. On several occasions, following lawn-bowling tournaments, I found him comatose and would wait hours for his return to consciousness. At such times, he couldn't remember events leading up to his drunken stupor. His business was slipping away and his wife was desperate.

The episode of the unsuccessful trip to the Bell Clinic taught me never again to send a patient for treatment while he was still drinking. Thereafter I always waited for the drunk to sober up. I should have downgraded my interest in the drug alcohol and probed more deeply into this intelligent man's overuse to understand his reasons for drinking. What meaning did life have for him after his mid-years? How important was success and why was he so little disturbed by accelerating failure? What a person believes is reality. For him nothing else is real, even if the rest of us find his beliefs bizarre and ridiculous.

Am I an alcoholic? This is frequently asked of a family doctor. In turn, I often tossed the question back to the patient: "Do you think you are an alcoholic?" After discussion I might say, "You decide." Such self-decisions by patients have special therapy values. A realtor so challenged promptly decided to test himself. He was particularly worried about his urgent need for a couple of cocktails at the beginning of every social gathering before he could begin to enjoy himself. He resolved on his own to set aside the month of January annually as a period of complete abstinence from both alcohol and smoking. In a couple of years he found he could easily dispense with all smoking. Though I don't know the long-term effect of his annual month of abstinence from alcohol, I do know it had a salutary temporary effect. He was amazed and delighted to note how enjoyable each January could be without the aid of liquor.

Arthur, though a few years younger than I, was one of my closest friends. In the twenties and thirties he was a confirmed alcoholic—and in the fifties he was cured. By that I mean that he learned to control his excessive drinking, to limit himself to beer at intervals and to ardent spirits occasionally. He appeared to fear the latter, though he never admitted it. In curbing his overuse of alcohol, he learned an acceptable pattern of social drinking. Some may say that Arthur had never been an alcoholic. In my books he was a full-blown one, because he drank compulsively, was often deeply intoxicated. Furthermore, he had frequent blackouts.

How many alcoholics cure themselves? Two surveys at an interval of ten years by the Addiction Research Foundation of Ontario in Frontenac County suggest that nearly twenty-five per cent do. One active treatment authority estimates that up to five per cent may do so. I have the greatest respect for Alcoholics Anonymous because that organization has done more for alcoholics than any other group, and one of its basic tenets is: "Once an alcoholic, always an alcoholic." In the experience of the organization there are no assured cures.

In treating problem drinkers I wouldn't use the prospect of complete cure as a major inducement for abstinence, but surely in the name of truth and honesty these people should know that there is a very slight prospect of moderate social drinking again after five years or so of complete abstinence. Nothing is ever gained by making the future gloomier than the facts warrant.

What resources did my friend Arthur draw upon in mastering his overuse of alcohol? I do not know. Probably the understanding and complete loyalty of his wife was a major factor. Perhaps I helped a little. I know I tried. If I succeeded, he was the only addict among my patients whom I rehabilitated. This, over a period of thirty years, is not a record to be proud of.

Cecil was one of the ablest salesmen-merchants I have met. Before "Honest Ed" came on the scene in Toronto, Cecil had adopted his methods, though on a smaller scale. Every cubic foot of his store was filled with merchandise with the price clearly marked on each item. This was in his later life. As a young man in British Columbia he had been an advanced alcoholic with long benders of six weeks or more in a hotel three or four times a year, ending with medical attention in hospital. In mid-life he had fallen in love with a fine intelligent woman who consented to marriage if he gave up alcohol. He kept his promise through a successful marriage to the age of eighty-four years.

The lesson to be drawn from this is that we can do the most difficult things if the pay-off is great enough. Many a smoker has been able to give up smoking after persuading himself wherein it will be worthwhile.

Industry in Ontario with its program of so-called "constructive coercion" is learning how to help early problem-drinker employees. They must take treatment *as a condition of continuing employment.* Some programs are getting 60 to 70 per cent cure rates, higher than those of most alcoholism clinics. I have sometimes wondered how written contracts between problem drinkers and their doctors would work. In the contract the patient would agree to abstinence for a certain period—or else the doctor wouldn't attend him any longer. It is worth trying.

Another respected merchant permitted considerable drinking in his home and shared in it. He had three sons who were all bright fellows. The eldest was in his late thirties when I was asked for help. About three times a year he would go on a six-week bender, leaving his wife to manage the store. During one of these benders I put him in hospital. In two days he was enjoying his meals again, but complained of hearing the nurses talking about him in the corridor. I explained that this was an hallucination and probably a precursor to the D.T.'s. As I intended, this greatly alarmed him. After several days he stopped hearing voices and was discharged from hospital. Subsequently, he got in touch with Brigadier Monk of the Salvation Army in Toronto and ceased drinking.

This man taught me several things. He was the first patient with acute intoxication whom I treated with intravenous glucose. I learned this therapy (which is now outdated) in a few hours with Dr. Gordon Bell. It was immensely gratifying to see the patient resume eating in a couple of days. With the earlier treatment of sedation and forcing fluids by mouth it might take six days for the patient to regain his appetite. Also, this man made me realize that I was a failure as a mental-health helper or psychotherapist. I couldn't get either him or his wife to confide in me about the drinking problem. The fact that the Salvation Army promptly led him into a life of sobriety deflated me and I was envious.

The second brother in this family was an incorrigible alcoholic. He showed no interest whatever in controlling his consumption of liquor and seemed quite satisfied to live in the contracted world of the habitual drinker. Some might say that these two brothers owed their addictions to the permissive attitude that prevailed in the home. This is too simple a deduction as a third son was a complete abstainer.

The medical profession should be able to do more for the over-user of alcohol than any other group because it has more going for it. Why hasn't it? It hasn't, I believe, because it has neglected to include the study of alcoholism in medical school curricula and because there is a paucity of refresher courses for family doctors by authorities speaking their language.

One of the most fetching alcoholics I ever met had been addicted all his adult life. A graduate engineer, he held a responsible position, raised and educated a fine family of three children. After retirement at sixty-five he continued with periodic bouts of excessive drinking and eventually, unable to get car-accident insurance, lost his driver's permit because of irresponsible driving. One of his first thoughts on each sobering-up was to encircle a date on the calendar for the next period of intoxication to begin. His life of periodic inebriation was carefully planned. He must have thought he was getting something pretty valuable out of it. What was it?

It was in 1916 that Premier Hearst's government brought in the Ontario Temperance Act (OTA) forbidding the purchase of alcoholic beverages except for industrial, religious and medical purposes. The act was repealed under Premier Ferguson in 1927. This Ontario prohibition period of eleven years is not easy to forget.

Doctors were permitted to sign prescriptions for alcohol and I signed six to ten per week for a fee of one dollar each. They were all for six ounces of whiskey. All kinds of excuses and subterfuges were used to obtain a prescription: diarrhaea, rheumatism and heart trouble were favorite complaints. I remember a Windsor physician reporting that in one week he had no less than two hundred whiskey seekers, including twelve women.

Whatever else this era of Prohibition did, it degraded the physicians of our province by making them virtually bartenders and bootleggers. The citizens lost a measure of respect for their doctors.

Some of the effects of Prohibition were terrifying. Many young men learned to drink excessively because it was forbidden and thereby the smart thing to do. I recollect two boys in their late teens whose stomachs on separate occasions I pumped out in hay mows. One was in the loft of the local town hostler who kept horses for rental. The other was in a farm barn. Both boys wanted to keep their intoxicated state unknown to others.

I soon abandoned the stomach-washing procedure as ineffective, for usually by the time I saw the patient there was little alcohol in the stomach. Then I tried apomorphine hypodermics, which caused prompt and vigorous vomiting. However, this made the patient appear and feel very ill. I early discarded this treatment as being too drastic.

Other serious results of Prohibition were that it allowed the bootlegger with his more dangerous products to flourish and it also prompted the habitual drinker to turn for thirst quenchers to such products as rubbing alcohol which is poisonous methyl alcohol.

Wild Bill MacPherson was so accurately labelled by his nickname that I feared him. He appeared in my office at eleven o'clock one Saturday night in the midst of a three-day blizzard.

"I want a prescription for six ounces of alcohol," he announced. "The druggist will give me a bottle of rubbing alcohol for it."

I knew he could drink a bottle of rubbing alcohol at one sitting with little or no apparent ill effects.

I refused. "No, William. How will you get the fifteen miles

home tonight by horse and cutter in a storm like this? Moreover, the two pharmacists are closed."

He picked up my prescription pad and wrote: "Wild Bill MacPherson needs 6 ounces of whiskey."

"Now Doctor, sign."

Sunday morning I found an empty bottle labelled Rubbing Alcohol on my waiting-room table. He proved his point.

In many ways Wild Bill was quite a person. As well as being rugged, wild and unpredictable when drinking, which was often, he had a heart of gold where his family was concerned. That same winter his son—a long, lean, lanky fellow of twenty—was seriously ill with pneumonia.

"Doctor, would a little whiskey help?" Wild Bill wanted to know.

"Perhaps. It certainly won't harm him and it might relax him."

"If you give me a prescription I won't take a drop."

I did, and he was as good as his word. The boy recovered. This was before the days of penicillin when we tried all the supportive measures we could think of for pneumonia.

The emotionally disturbed, the suicides, the narcotic addicts and excessive drinkers: they all have something in common in that their compulsions lead them toward self-destruction. I didn't often understand them but I found many of them interesting as people and fascinating subjects for study.

VI. "Everywhere the Old Order Changes . . ."

As the decade of the twenties merged into the thirties it heralded a time of change. The depression which began in 1929 was to alter life in many ways. Militarism was building up in Europe, soon to cast its shadow over the Western hemisphere. And the revolution in therapeutic medicine, just around the corner, would transform medical practices in ways no one could foresee. A whole new world was in the making.

Somewhere Sir William Osler has said, "Everywhere the old order changes, and happy is he who changes with it." For the first seven years of practice, I didn't go anywhere for refresher courses. Establishing a practice was like tending a baby; the younger it was, the more close care it needed. Like many of my colleagues, I was spending about a hundred dollars a year on medical books, but I felt I was not getting enough continuing education because the practice stopped increasing.

It seemed obvious that I must study more. One cannot stand still; it was as simple as that. On consultation with my wife it was decided that we would take an annual holiday in a city in the late summer; we were seeing enough of the country the rest of the year. We chose Chicago for its Cook County Hospital and New York for the Polyclinic, reasoning that I could spend every morning attending postgraduate classes, with the afternoons and evenings free for entertainment and relaxation.

For a modest fee of twenty dollars the Cook County Hospital postgraduate school offered a full two-week program of clinics, discussions, and demonstrations. One year it was ear-nose-and-throat studies. Another, it was rectal troubles, then children's diseases, etc. In a few years it was both surprising and gratifying to note how much new medicine had been covered. Best of all, the practice soon began to expand again and my patients developed a lively interest in my refresher program, wanting to know about the next holiday and course of study. These annual working holidays, which helped keep me abreast of the times, became an obvious and natural pattern of my life.

With the passing of years I eventually became dissatisfied with my limited office facilities and in 1937 alterations were made to the building which allowed for two more examining rooms, a surgery, enlarged laboratory with storage space and a dark room for developing X-ray film. This modest extension coincided with a remarkable expansion of diagnostic and therapeutic aids available for the first time to the general practitioner. A mere recital of these indicates how the face of medicine was changing for the family doctor.

The therapeutic revolution, which brought a whole new arsenal of drugs to medicine, occurred between the years 1930 and 1950. The first of the miracle drugs for infections appeared in 1932 with the introduction of Prontosil. This was followed in 1937 by sulfanilamide and Dagenan (sulfapyridine).

It was about 1937 that the Quartz Lamp appeared. Though of limited application, it was a great help to patients with some forms of eczema. I found it a godsend in healing lesions caused by the horrible affliction of *pruritus ani.*

The portable X-ray was introduced for home and office use and produced excellent film of limbs, spine, pelvis, chest, and skull of a quality acceptable to the Workmen's Compensation Board.

The Sandorn Cardiette, an electrocardiograph machine housed in a case small enough to be easily carried, became available in the mid-1930's. It was a boon to a general practitioner practicing at a distance from a heart specialist, provided he was trained to interpret its tracings.

Diathermy machines with their heating pads were offered about 1937 by medical supply houses. They were helpful in many ways, particularly in giving relief to patients with sinus infections. These machines had electronic coagulation equipment permitting excision of lesions, such as small skin cancers. I used them extensively on early skin cancer and it was very rare to see a recurrence.

Obtaining and using all this range of equipment in my enlarged quarters was in no sense out of the ordinary. Hundreds of Ontario family physicians at this time were doing the same thing. What is amazing is that so many advances for the family doctor came to hand at one time—so many that the year 1937 was an important milepost for the profession, despite the fact that it was an uneasy period in general. The depression had not yet run its course, and on the international scene this was the year when Stalin's purges were at their height. More than half the 1936 members of the Soviet Congress had been arrested for counter-revolutionary moves. The head of the Ukrainian Party was liquidated after saying simply that he didn't believe the many who had been faithful for so long had suddenly become traitors.

About this time Ontario general practitioners were deep in another experiment—that of working together in partnerships and groups. In 1936 I engaged an assistant doctor who had just completed his hospital internship, and the association was so successful that I soon concluded never again to practice alone if I could avoid it. A helper gave me relief from duty on occasional evenings, week-ends and holidays.

It is curious how excessive devotion to interesting work can come to have all the elements of an addiction. The alcoholic, while under the influence of alcohol, thinks he is having a wonderful time in his own little world. In the same way, a physician can build a complete world around patient activities and shut out his own family and his own adequate health care. This was happening to me in the mid-thirties, with my wife carrying too much of the upbringing of my children.

I had to develop techniques for working with a partner. From 1938 onwards, an assistant or associate was hired annually through the superintendent or chief-of-staff of a large city hospital. The salary in the beginning was $100 a month, rising after a few years to $150, sometimes with board and the use of a car. We had no written contract. Each agreement was verbal and could be terminated by either of us on a month's notice. Some may call this a poor business arrangement, but it worked—except for a period during World War II when I couldn't get an assistant for three years. There was no stipulation as to where these helpers could practice on leaving me. In telling them that they could hang their hat next door at any time, I wasn't as brave as I appeared. I simply believed that this was probably the best way to keep them away from my territory.

All seriously ill patients were seen by both of us. All maternity patients under the care of one of us had to be examined by the other at least once. This ensured that if the doctor engaged for the confinement was unavailable when needed, the other could take over.

I always called my helper an associate, never an assistant. I made it clear to each that there was only one thing I would not forgive him for, and that was criticising or cutting me down behind my back. He must be loyal to me as I would be to him. This was not intended to condone mistakes because we must be completely candid in discussing patients and their therapy. It was simply a necessary basis for working together.

The depression years were a harrowing experience. Officially, in Canada, the depression began with the stock market crash on Tuesday, October 29, 1929, and ended September 1, 1939, when Hitler invaded Poland. It mentally scarred most doctors of that day for they were never able thereafter to cast aside feelings of skepticism and doubt about the soundness of the country's economy, no matter how healthy and flourishing it might appear to be—another depression just might occur.

As to how I fared financially—my gross income in 1929 was $6,600; four years later in 1933, which was the bottom of the depression in Ontario, the annual receipts had shrunk by one-third to $4,400. This was very serious, because the decrease represented all the profits. Fortunately, by this time I owned my car and most of my house and equipment. The furnace had been changed from coal back to wood. The depression reached the point where it was futile to send accounts to former good-paying patients. I was collecting only 60 per cent of my fees and, worst of all, I was charging less. The lower the fees, the more likely it was the patient would try to pay, or so it seemed. Employment was at a low ebb and many families in the village were on relief. The farmers were a little better off in that they had their own milk, eggs, meat, and vegetables. They were happy to barter for our services. Farm produce and more wood for the furnace than we could either use or store were offered in payment of accounts.

In regard to my income, I might add that never in my thirty years of practice was I able to add more than a thousand dollars to my worth a year. I resented paying so much income tax because it thwarted me from building an old-age security or reasonable retirement fund. And it disturbed me to read the annual reports from Ottawa giving doctors' incomes as the highest professional incomes in Canada. They were higher than my own. The only really wealthy family doctors I knew had either made a killing in the stock market, or had inherited a fair fortune, or married a wealthy woman.

The one time I ventured into the stock market I did so timidly. It was in 1933, when for reasons I cannot recall I borrowed $1000 at a local bank and invested it in General Motors stock at $24.00 a share. I sold it in a year when it had doubled in value and I never went back into the market. Why? Because I found myself looking first at the stock-market page every morning. Had I held on to these shares until 1960, someone has estimated, my original investment would have been worth $17,000. My only conclusion from this is that I was a poor business man. I didn't spend enough time counting money. However, my regrets are few. My work brought compensations that outweighed monetary ones by far.

The depression, for all its evil effects, had a way of bringing people together. We were all struggling to survive and such differences as there were between us were minimized. Today there is debate about how much and in what way the needy poor should receive help from society. There is considerable friction between the givers and receivers of welfare, which creates a strangely different atmosphere from that of the twenties and thirties. I doubt if then either the doctors or their needy patients looked upon the completely indigent as "charity" cases. Rather, we took their existence as a fact of life, a necessary condition for living with our neighbors. A person paid if he could. The doctors didn't seem to be unduly unhappy contributing services on occasion and the poor reciprocated with appreciation, by not making unreasonable demands.

During these years also, through community ventures not strictly medical in nature, I was forming associations that were among the most pleasant features of my stay in Lucknow. There was the independent group calling themselves The Clansmen, a local service organization that refused affiliation with international bodies like the Lions and Rotary Clubs. The Clansmen limited membership to twenty, although one year it went up to thirty-five. They were nearly all young business men, of varied talents which they used generously in the promotion of worthy local projects. I was constantly amazed at their ability to relate successfully to all kinds of people, to act effectively in public meetings and to analyze social situations. I could discuss any public health matter with them and get results. With little argument the club agreed to pay for eyeglasses for all school children in the area who needed them. They cooperated fully with local groups of national organizations such as the Canadian Cancer Society and the Ontario Tuberculosis Association. I admired these young men and concluded that there really wasn't as much difference between doctors and other citizens as is often imagined; we were all "parts of one another."

This service club had some major accomplishments to its credit. It bought the Officers' Mess Quarters of the large Port

Albert Airport and moved it to Lucknow to serve as a community hall. It started a hockey arena. And one winter the Lucknow young men set up a sort of open forum for discussion of timely social issues. Meeting every Sunday in the United Church Auditorium, they would listen to some authority propound his subject followed by an open discussion. Speakers included a prominent dentist, a city police chief, an RCMP officer and the Mayor of Toronto. We invited Tim Buck, the head of the Canadian Communist party, to address us but this invitation didn't sit well with some of the church fathers. The situation was saved by Tim Buck writing that a previous engagement prevented him from accepting.

As the years went on, medical group activities also took toll of my time. The Bruce County Medical Society met annually, and that of Huron County at longer intervals. The meetings were usually addressed by a university medical teacher discussing a timely subject and I always made an effort to attend. In later years I became district representative to the Council of the Ontario Medical Association, an activity which so interested me that I became more and more involved in the business of the OMA and was made president for the year 1949-50.

This called for considerable absence from my practice and it was interesting to see how my colleagues reacted. I mean this. Most of them returned the patients I regularly cared for whom they had attended in my absence, but an appreciable number never did. I didn't discuss this with them, leaving it entirely to their own discretion and judgment.

Though difficult in many ways, this period of transition following my first decade of practice—when therapeutic medicine was taking on a new face and the world was hurtling from depression into war—was a time too of learning and growing. The changes going on were not always perceptible but in small ways we were moving toward dramatic changes to come.

VII. A Time of Revolution

With the advent of sulfa drugs in the thirties the therapeutic revolution was well under way. As I have said, they put an end to such severe tissue infections as that of Annie's finger and erysipelas; quinsies melted away, running ears quickly dried up, mastoid operations became almost a surgeon's lost art, rheumatic fever dwindled, bacterial endocarditis was no longer an implacable death sentence and child-bed fever disappeared as a threat to mothers.

Sulfanilamide, its many compounds and derivatives, came in the beginning from dyes. One was a brick-red dye called Prontosil. Dr. Gerhard Domagk, a physician with the German dye industry, in a search for anti-germ substances injected the compound into mice infected with streptococcus germs—whereupon the mice turned a brilliant red but recovered from the infection. This was in 1932. The following year Prontosil was injected into a ten-month-old infant with a staphylococcus infection. The child promptly recovered. Other experimentation followed and in 1937 two American physicians, Doctors Perrin Long and Eleanor Bliss, gave it to a seven-year-old child with erysipelas. In twelve hours the child's temperature was normal. When next it was given to a woman dangerously ill with child-bed fever, her temperature too returned to normal overnight.

Prontosil was a patented drug. The brilliant work of French chemists at the Pasteur Institute broke this dye molecule into two parts. The dye part was medically useless; the powerful germ-killing properties residing in the remaining part were identified as sulfanilamide, a compound which had been synthesized in 1908 but was forgotten because it had no known use. It now appeared on the market as a quick successor to Prontosil.

Since 1937 more than five thousand sulfa drugs have been synthesized by universities, institutes, pharmaceutical laboratories, etc. Most of them were useless, but a dozen or so have transformed the medical treatment of infections. And among the chief beneficiaries were the children being born into a safer world.

Carefully kept records show that in my thirty years of practice I attended 1100 confinements and had one maternal death; three deliveries in one day and sixty-five in one year were the maximum. This was not a large maternity practice. Many general practitioners were attending several hundred maternity patients a year. My area people were not that prolific. That I had but one maternal death was, I think, a creditable record but not especially so. I may have met with an unusually small number of serious complications. Whether this is so or not, I dislike drawing conclusions from small numbers, having in mind the story of a lumber camp in northern Quebec staffed by 50 lumberjacks and 2 women cooks. When one of the loggers seduced one of the cooks the statistics showed that 50 per cent of the women had been seduced by 2 percent of the men. Which is rather ridiculous, of course! Conclusions from small numbers are untrustworthy. Nevertheless, I think I may conclude from my record that I didn't commit many errors of commission. I had one birth by Caesarean section, a record I would have difficulty defending as I do not know if there were any babies damaged or lost from too long a labor. I do recall two women who refused to become pregnant again because of long painful first labors. These probably should have had their births by Caesarean section.

Bringing life into the world has always been fraught with hazard—and may always be. Among the hazards, so-called "crib deaths" have long defied explanation. They are invariably unexpected, striking down seemingly healthy infants when they are asleep in their cribs—hence the name. Statistics are not trustworthy because police often attribute such deaths to suffocation or respiratory infection, but it has been estimated that about 1 in 300 infants born in the United States die in this way. I saw at least a dozen in my practice, and one of the earliest was the baby of the only mother I lost in confinement.

The woman and her husband were recent arrivals from Germany after his discharge from the army following World War I. It wasn't a complicated pregnancy, but I hadn't paid enough attention to a sudden gush of blood, about a half cup, at six and a half months. This usually means a placenta placed too close to the mouth of the womb. The woman's labor was normal. There was no difficulty, except that the placenta didn't seem to want to come away. So I removed it carefully manually—and went home. I was recalled two hours later to find the woman dead from a sudden massive hemorrhage. An autopsy at once revealed that there was no tear of the womb but its lower portion was as thin as paper. Never again did I remove an after-birth manually. If it was delayed, I would attach a small weight to the cord and leave the mother to be watched for bleeding until I could return.

In the days following the mother's death the baby seemed to thrive. It was plump and healthy looking. Then in two weeks it was found dead in its crib one morning.

The grief-stricken father left the community after the double tragedy, with these parting words to me: "I've had enough of this country. I'm going home to Düsseldorf." I couldn't blame him.

Another early crib death was unusual for a different reason. A Mr. A. came in late on a Saturday evening to ask for his account, saying, "I want to pay it."

The account went back for more than a year and included services for a confinement which had gone well.

"It is $64.50," I told him.

"Make out a cheque," A. said, then interrupted himself. "Just a minute. I've been told that it is unlucky to pay the whole of a doctor's bill. Perhaps I should leave a dollar owing."

"Do as you please," I agreed.

"No. Make it out in full."

I did so and he left.

Next morning at daybreak I had a frantic call from him. The baby was dead in its crib. Mere coincidence or chance make bedfellows of unrelated incidents and circumstances.

At one period in the early 1930's these deaths were being called thymic deaths. Behind the thyroid gland in our neck is a small thymus gland which, when swollen, was supposed to cause lethal pressure damage. X-raying the neck would reduce its size. I referred all newborn babies, at that period, to a London hospital for X-ray of their thymus glands to prevent the possibility of crib death. This procedure, however, was abandoned by the medical profession as ineffective after two years. Now the thinking is that there are many causes contributing to such infant deaths, including overwhelming infections such as the pneumonias, cardiac arrest, allergic shock, some hormone deficiencies, laryngeal spasm and even smothering. With modern drugs and techniques and this new awareness, it is possible to anticipate trouble areas and prevent many of these deaths from happening.

One Toronto mother lost three children from crib death and a fourth was being carefully watched for cardiac arrest when she admitted to smothering all the former children.

It may be added that these crib deaths of unknown cause have no geographic boundaries. About the same death rate has been found wherever studies have been made, from Belfast to Prague to Manila. A long-term study needs to be done to determine why the disease occurs at certain ages and not at others. It does not strike babies in the first few days of life and is rare after six months. As recently as 1972, an outbreak of crib deaths in New York has drawn attention to this baffling ailment and stimulated more intensive research into its causes.

Another infant problem yielded miraculously to the scientific advances of the thirties. Uncontrolled spontaneous bleeding of the newborn, affecting both sexes equally, has plagued medical science for centuries. The severity of the condition varies widely. Sometimes bleeding is so slight it is no more than an inconvenience, but in other instances it is so acute that death results. Hemorrhages may come from the navel cord, palate, skin or any internal organ, with bleeding into the brain particularly dangerous. Because of this predisposed blood deficiency in infants, the Jews years ago postponed to the eighth day the circumcision of their boy infants.

Authorities differ concerning the number of babies who are predisposed to this hemorrhaging. Some say that 1 in 500 is in danger. Others insist that this figure is two or three times higher. I saw about ten of them, with two deaths. The accepted treatment was fresh blood transfusions which probably came into vogue at the end of the First World War. On one matter there is unanimous agreement. Small premature babies are in special danger of suffering death or permanent injury as a result of this bleeding.

Then in 1939, with the discovery of Vitamin K, the whole picture changed and another disease was conquered. Vitamin K is now given to the mother before confinement, or to the newborn infant, or to both. It is a perfect preventive measure.

Vitamins are substances found in certain foods in trace amounts which are essential to maintain life but do not themselves supply energy. More than forty have been identified and they are named after letters of the alphabet.

The story of the discovery of Vitamin K is a strange and complex one.* A triad of major researchers contributed. The first one to be heard from was Henrik Dam, Assistant Professor at the University of Copenhagen. He knew that laboratory baby chicks are in danger of bleeding to death from small wounds because their blood fails to clot and even when drawn off may fail to coagulate. Henrik Dam in the early 1930's decided to try and find out more about the digestive processes of domestic fowl as a preliminary to knowing more about bleeding chicks.

He began by giving one hundred laboratory chicks a ration which the knowledge of that day affirmed was balanced for healthy growth. It included pure fats, starches, proteins and all

* Cf. Webb Garrison, "Vitamin K, Savior of Bleeding Babies", *Today's Health* (September 1969), 42.

the known vitamins. In a couple of weeks the chicks were oozing blood into their pinfeathers, followed by hemorrhages into their muscles and body cavities. After six weeks only three of the 100 were alive and these were scarcely able to wobble about.

Dam concluded there was no infection and that there must be something important lacking in their diet. He supplemented their ration by adding fruits and vegetables which made no difference. However, giving certain cereals and seeds dramatically stopped the bleeding. He continued his experiments and by 1935 he knew that the factor preventing the chicks bleeding was found also in alfalfa, outer cabbage leaves and spinach.

Dam at first didn't know what to call the unknown anti-hemorrhage factor and then named it Koagulationsvitamine. The Anglo-Saxon world didn't accept this heavy-handed name and labelled it Vitamin K.

The second major researcher appeared on the scene. A group of English research workers headed by W. D. McFarlane, without any knowledge of Dam's work, began to puzzle out why identification bands inserted into the wings of laboratory birds made small wounds that bled for hours. They fed putrid fish meal to some of their chicks and the bleeding stopped at once. They concluded their blood-clotting substance was the product of germ activity.

Independent scientists concluded that the findings of both these researches were sound and that there must be at least two blood-clotting substances. One is found in green plants and was tentatively called Vitamin K-1 while the other is produced by bacteria and was called Vitamin K-2.

The problem remained of isolating the blood clotting agent and then finding out exactly what it was and also, if possible, to produce it synthetically. A number of research chemists attempted this.

And here is where the last of the triad of major researchers comes in. At St. Louis University Edward A. Doisy began extracting it from alfalfa. He knew that Vitamin K was widely found in nature but in concentrations that were very low—so low that it would be a costly investigation. He asked the university and other backers for money and tons and tons of alfalfa. After spending nearly $200,000, he isolated small quantities of a yellow oil which was almost pure Vitamin K. Then he produced in the laboratory a chemical with blood-clotting properties similar to the natural Vitamin K. Doisy completed his work and patented it in 1939-40.

In the spring of 1939 Dr. William W. Waddell Jr., Professor of Pediatrics of the University of Virginia School of Medicine, was the first doctor who courageously authorized the injection of Vitamin K into a bleeding baby. The bleeding stopped in a few hours and the infant was at home quite well in a few days.

Soon physicians were hailing Vitamin K as one of the miracle drugs. Chewing gum and aspirin enriched with the vitamin were put on the market. As with most new discoveries there were a few doctors who were over enthusiastic. Employing too large doses, they found these had some harmful side effects. The trend now is to protect all newborn babies from spontaneous bleeding by giving the vitamin to expectant mothers or to the infants or to both.

If another member is born to your family, it is almost certain the vitamin will be used, though your doctor may not tell you as its use is often by routine order to the hospital staff. Its use is estimated to save the lives of at least 5000 babies a year in the United States and this indicates that probably 500 are saved annually in Canada.

Incidentally, it took only a few tests to find that Vitamin K (natural or synthetic) is ineffective with hemophilia, the hereditory bleeding disease.

One of the strangest quirks of the whole story of Vitamin K discovery is that the initial researcher Henrik Dam chose to study the nutrition of baby chicks. If he had selected animals usually used in research such as guinea pigs, mice, dogs, rabbits, etc., he would never have discovered the existence of Vitamin K. All fowl including mature hens and roosters as well as baby chicks are in danger of bleeding to death and must receive Vitamin K as a dietary factor, which they do from cereals and seeds. But this isn't true of mammals because soon after birth they obtain Vitamin K as a by-product of bacterial action in their bowel.

As early as the 1880's scientists drew attention to the fact that the bowels and colons of all human adults are teeming with germs while the gut of newborn babies is sterile, but they didn't know the significance of this difference. Now it appears that one of the by-products of our bowel micro-organisms is to provide us with Vitamin K and the newborn baby doesn't get this required amount of Vitamin K until his gut becomes plentifully inhabited by germs and bacteria.

And still another mystery has been cleared up. Early in this century some doctors reported that babies with hemorrhagic disease of the newborn who were of well-to-do parents, born in hospitals and kept for some days in sterile nurseries seemed to bleed longer than those born in homes and in unsanitary surroundings teeming with germs. It seems reasonable now to conclude that the babies of the poor were obtaining their colonies of gut germs earlier and hence were building their reserves of Vitamin K faster. Apparently all advantages of the good life in our society do not rest with the affluent.

The jaundiced newborn was also with us throughout my practicing days, and that condition too was greatly ameliorated by discoveries attending the therapeutic revolution. I am using the old name of this ailment. Some of the babies so afflicted got better, though many died and we didn't know why. As a result, we did a lot of silent praying. I recall one young mother whose first baby was deeply jaundiced and was sent to London hospital where it was saved by blood transfusions. The mother's second baby was also jaundiced. This was in the mid-1930's.

Until the late twenties, as many as 50 per cent of the jaundiced newborn died or were left with brain damage. The jaundice caused the brain damage. Then it was discovered that replacing all the infant's blood with fresh blood got rid of the jaundice. The first replacement transfusion in Toronto was in 1927. Replacement transfusions after this became standard treatment and the mortality rate dropped to about 5 per cent.

The government assisted by making available certain hospitals in Ontario as centers for such transfusions.

It was a great advance when, in 1940, the Rh blood groups were discovered. The disease was then given the name *Erythroblastosis fetalis*, or if the baby's anemia rather than the jaundice was a prominent feature it was termed *Icterus gravis neonatorum*. This latter is a hemolysis of the infant's red blood cells due to the presence of the anti-Rh agglutinins in the mother's serum. These antibodies develop *in utero*, in the presence of an RH positive fetus, and result in anemia.

Following the discovery of the Rh factor, it became possible for physicians to recognize the mother about to give birth to a jaundiced baby. Many family doctors now send their maternity patients, when first interviewed, into hospital for tests to determine their blood grouping and the presence of blood antibodies. If the latter indicates that the patient is Rh negative, she is given further tests before the thirty-fourth week. Antibody levels are thereby watched, the woman likely to give birth to a jaundiced baby is identified and her doctor is thus alerted well in advance of the confinement.

About the time the Rh factor was discovered there was an important development in therapeutic techniques affecting the health of the very young.

In the mid-twenties the diarrheal diseases were the commonest cause of children's deaths, particularly in their second year. Acute intestinal intoxication could occur at any time, but it was most prevalent in the late summer and autumn. Sometimes called *cholera morbus* and *cholera infantum*—names which had no connection with the epidemic Asiatic cholera—the disease was marked by a dull and listless appearance, dry ashy skin and sunken eyes, persistent vomiting and profuse watery diarrhea. It could come on with alarming rapidity in one or two days and end in death within another twenty-four hours.

Although this illness has not been finally conquered, and is still serious in some areas, it was a red-letter day when about 1940 we learned how to revive our young patients and start them on the road to recovery by injecting fluids under the skin of the abdomen and axillae.

The newborn was assuredly coming into a much safer world.

Attention to teeth as a major seat of infection and bodily ills was one of the things which changed the character of medical practice in the thirties and forties.

In the 1920's we rarely saw children with a full set of teeth, a chief reason being that dental care was unheard of. As in my own youth, a bothersome tooth was pulled; the cavity wasn't filled. But awareness was growing, and in 1939 the people of Lucknow district started a program of tooth care for all their public-school children. In that year the village and two townships engaged the services of the local dentist, Dr. James Little, to examine and treat every child in his office at least once a year. Later another township came into the scheme. The government paid one-third of the cost and in time, as I remember, this assistance was increased to one-half. This was one of the first such programs in Ontario, if not the first.

Dr. Little estimated that 800 children, aged six to fourteen years, were being checked annually. It gave him care of the first permanent teeth—the so-called six-year molars. He recalls that "there were only two or three young rebels among the lot"—one of these fled his office and locked himself in the family car. A county public-health nurse reported an astonishing improvement in the children's mouths. In the beginning as many as eight cavities per child was not unusual. After only two years' care figures showed, on an average, one cavity per two children.

On instituting this program of public health care, it was interesting that many of the more affluent village families refused any part of it. With their rugged individualism they wanted no financial aid whatever, from government or municipality. Finally, however, they agreed to share in it, largely because it was easier to operate the program that way.

For public health in general, the program was a giant step forward.

The revolution in the treatment of fractures over the past thirty years has been one of the marked advances in my time. I can't possibly deal adequately here with the many types of fractures we saw, but a few examples will suggest some of the new and improved treatments that were coming into vogue during the thirties and on into the forties.

Fractures were common among my people as farming is one of the most hazardous of occupations.

One extraordinary incident though it did not involve a fracture, reveals what peculiar accidents can take place on a farm.

A hurry-up call to a house on a July afternoon found me looking at a middle-aged man lying comfortably on the lawn after being lifted off a rod which had impaled him through his chest.

He had been repairing his windmill which had a main driving rod consisting of two rods locked together end to end about six feet above the ground. He had unlocked these rods while he worked on a temporary platform above the end of the exposed lower rod. The platform collapsed dropping him onto the rod. Its end had entered the lower part of his neck in front just above the notch in the upper edge of the chest bone and had come out of his back between a shoulder blade and the spine. He was impaled on the rod like a chicken on a spit.

A neighbor courageously had lifted him off the rod. I accompanied the injured man in an ambulance to Goderich hospital 20 miles away. I felt surely he must have some internal chest injuries, but he insisted he was comfortable. His only request was for a smoke.

The entry and exit made by the rod were bleeding a little and, of course, were dressed. A chest X-ray showed that the rod had gone through the top portion of a lung. He required no further attention and went home in a week quite well.

The end of the rod was about one inch by a half inch with rounded edges. Apparently on its passage through the chest, it had pushed the gullet and vital blood vessels to one side. He was a fortunate man indeed to get off so lightly from such an accident.

In my early days of practice the community seemed always to have a couple of humpbacks who owed their disability to untreated spinal fractures. And there was one peg-leg in the village—the knee joint fixed at a right angle, due probably to inflammation rather than to a fracture though a fracture may have been involved.

Margaret, a spinster of eighty years, tiny and thin, fell off the back stoop of her house and injured her hip. While I was carrying her into the house she tried to lighten the occasion by quipping, "I wish you to know, Doctor, that you are the first man ever to roll down my stockings." Her thigh bone, the femur, appeared to be fractured. This was confirmed by my portable X-ray. Margaret didn't know how fortunate she was that the fracture occurred in the late 1940's rather than a few years earlier. Her hip bone was promptly pinned, she was encouraged to exercise in bed and in three months she was walking again. In the early 1930's she would have had a miserable time in bed for three months with a full-length leg cast suspended from a complicated framework over the bed and a weight attached to her leg. This treatment was very hazardous for elderly folk, with their chances of living through the first ten days rather slim.

In the early twenties a fracture of the shoulder or the upper end of the upper arm bone was also quite serious and the treatment of such an injury seems pretty cumbersome by today's standards. The patient was put to bed with the arm extended at right angles to the body and resting on a six-inch-wide board about five feet long. The trick was to make sure that the board was under the whole shoulder with its end reaching as far inward as the spine. Adhesive strips to the arm ended in a cord over a pulley with a weight on it. When the arm had been immobilized in this manner for six weeks the fracture would be healed. Though the arm bone always healed in good position, the treatment was an ordeal. Also, there was usually some resulting stiffness of the shoulder and elbow for several weeks from disuse.

Then in the 1930's we learned to treat this fracture by putting a pad in the axilla, binding the whole arm to the chest with the elbow in a flexed position. This procedure, particularly with elderly people, gave excellent results, and they could walk about while the fracture was healing.

Finally, in the 1940's, we found that all we had to do with this fracture of the upper end of the humerus was to put a cast on the arm from the wrist to the axilla with the elbow bent and the cast held by a sling around the neck, with the lower end of the sling attached to the wrist part of the cast. The weight of the cast kept the bone fragments in good position and they healed beautifully while the patient walked about or lay down as he pleased.

The modern treatment of a fractured ankle ushered in a new era. It was during the winter of 1940-41 when the reeve of our village, a man of my own age, fell and twisted his ankle. The portable X-ray showed a fracture. He was put to bed preparatory to putting on splints in a few days after the swelling had subsided. Then he would be forced to stay off the leg for five or six weeks.

I had just heard of a new treatment for fractures of this type. A telephone call to Dr. Roy Thomas, Chief of the Out-Patients Department of Toronto General Hospital, resulted in an invitation to go down and watch him treat fractures of the ankle in the new way. I did so. It was a wonder to watch him putting plaster-of-paris casts on the bare skin of the leg, incorporating in the cast a U-shaped iron with its closed end projecting from the bottom of the cast on which the patient would walk. The open legs of this walking iron were built into the cast. A few evenings later I put a similar cast on my friend's leg in his home on the kitchen table—leaving considerable plaster-of-paris on the floor for his wife to clean up, as she reminded me years later.

This little operation was the occasion for a party, probably to demonstrate the new treatment to the patient's friends who brought along some cheering ale for all of us. After a few weeks the cast was removed and my friend had excellent results.

Treating a fractured ankle with a skin-tight walking cast may not seem very exciting, but it was just about the most revolutionary medical treatment in my experience. I had been taught never to put fresh plaster-of-paris on the bare skin. It must always be over gauze or a dressing such as stockingette. I don't know what terrible things we thought would happen, though we did expect the hairs of the skin to be caught up in the plaster so that removal of the cast later would be painful. We soon learned that body hairs live only six weeks or less.

This was in 1940. From then on we put plaster-of-paris casts on the bare skin for many types of fractures. And a patient with a broken ankle was permitted to walk about while healing took place—a completely new idea.

It may seem strange that I applied the reeve's cast in the home rather than in the hospital. I rather liked working in patients' homes, not because I wanted to demonstrate any skills I might have but because there were distinct advantages. People talk more freely in familiar surroundings and their comments are often helpful, and the special assistance and facilities hospitals afford are frequently not really required. It was my way of counteracting, if only slightly, the unfortunate tendency to take medical care farther and farther away from the patient.

Among the major miseries of mankind today are a group of diseases under the name of arthritis. They include rheumathoid arthritis or just plain old-fashioned rheumatism and are especially troublesome for the middle-aged and elderly in the damp and cold months of the year. Little outstanding progress has been made in understanding them or providing relief from them although we do, of course, have aspirin and a drug called Butazolidin and cortisone to ease some of the aches and pains as well as physiotherapy programs to slow down their progressive ravages. One of the most terrible forms of this disease is arthritis of the spine, and for this some signal advances in treatment were made in the thirties and forties.

David was a healthy normal-appearing boy in a family of three children. He was all energy and seemed to fear nothing. A mischievous boy, he loved to knock flower pots from porches of women who he knew disliked him. As he grew into his early teens he seemed wiser than his years indicated. This was when disaster struck. He began to have pains in his back—at first mild, not severe enough for bed care. But it was soon apparent that something unusually serious was at work. The pains steadily became more severe and more widespread and, worst of all, he started to become stooped. The condition progressed so rapidly that in his early twenties the pain was unbearable without opiates and he was horribly misshapen with his body bent forward at right angles to his legs. It went on to kill him before he was thirty.

With his indomitable will he deserved a better fate. Long before his condition was fully developed he was in St. Michael's Hospital, Toronto, for a period of study. The consultant reported this conversation:

"David, I think you should spend a month in bed at home."

"What will that do for me?"

"It will ease the pain in your back."

"Will it cure me?"

"No, we do not know how to do that."

"Then I think I will die with my boots on."

It was early winter when he was in hospital. He was an ardent hockey fan and anxious to see the Maple Leafs play, but they wouldn't permit him to leave the hospital. So he raised the window, crawled out and shinnied down a drain pipe to the ground one floor below. With a pillow under his arm to sit on, he made his way to the arena a few blocks away. On his return he didn't think they had noted his absence.

David had what medical men know as ankylosing arthritis or *Arthritis deformans* of the spine. Its cause is unknown and there were no known measures in the 1920's to modify its ravages. A possible clue to the cause of David's ailment may be a fall he had in the school gymnasium while chinning himself on a ladder fastened horizontally to the ceiling of the room. He landed smack on his back on the cement floor six feet below and was knocked out for a few minutes, requiring a doctor to be summoned. I suggest that this severe trauma several months before the onset of his disease may have had something to do with precipitating it. But we don't know.

David was born twenty years too soon. In the early 1940's I had a second patient with this ailment, but what a different history he developed! By this time the medical profession had learned that if we kept the back straight all the time the arthritis would quieten down eventually, leaving the back rigid as a poker. The patient slept in a cast, wore a brace when up and about, and absented himself from work when he was tired. He was able to earn sufficient income as a carpenter to provide for his wife and two children. In time he led a surprisingly active life and you had to look closely to detect his stiff back.

This dramatic contrast between earlier and later methods of treating such spinal malfunctions also illustrates what a wonderful contribution surgeons have made without operating—just by more intelligent management.

In farming country years ago fires were also to be counted among the major hazards and the family doctor had to know a lot about treating burns.

Three children of the same farm family were playing with burning cattails which had been soaked in coal oil around a drum when it exploded. All were burned, but the lad who was astride the drum was in serious condition with second- and third-degree burns over most of his legs and hips.

This was in the mid-1920's. He was treated at home and in my office. At first the burned areas were cleaned with saline and weak Dakin's solution. When the slough was removed, snug dressings of vaseline and sometimes paraffin were applied, followed later near the end of healing by a scarlet red ointment. This was done daily. It took eight months to heal this boy's burns and another two weeks to get the stiffness out of his legs from the scar tissue. After that he was running about like any normal active lad.

About the same time, in the early 1920's, Dr. Murray Fisher of Gravenhurst was caring for a boy whose hands, legs and hips were badly burned from contact with high voltage wires. On the advice of Dr. R. Gaby, surgeon with the Ontario Hydro and reputed to be the best authority in Canada on electric burns, he dressed the boy's burns with gauze saturated with a mixture six-to-one of water and Hygeol, which is a chlorine product of

Wampole's. Then he applied snug bandages with elastoplast strips to help fill in the cavities and hurry skin formation. Dr. Fisher was delighted with the results.

Today the healing of the usual burns would be greatly hastened by skin grafting. Also, the doctors might paint the burned area with 0.5 percent silver nitrate and apply an ointment called Sulfamylon, which contains sulfanilamide and is bacteriostatic and bactericidal. General physicians in Toronto now are advised to use sterile dressings on small burns and to refer patients if more than 5 per cent of the body skin is burned.

Dr. E. K. Lyon of Leamington, Ontario, writing about his early treatment of burns, recalls that "tannic acid came into force about 1932 and was widely used for a period of about eight years, when it fell into disrepute. I was using skin grafting back in the late twenties and early thirties, but not the type of skin grafting we do today. It was done by the pinch graft method or sometimes by the Thiersch method, using postage-stamp grafts."

Treatment of burns with tannic acid has a long history. Thousands of years ago the Chinese were using tea leaves and the Jews were using ink. About 1930 the use of tannic acid was revived, first as a spray and then as a jelly and ointment. It fell into disrepute about 1940 because under the resulting crust, or eschar, abscesses would accumulate and also because a Dr. Wells demonstrated that it caused some liver and kidney damage.

Thiersch grafts were thin partial thickness grafts cut by hand. Then about 1936 the Pladgett dermatome appeared, cutting the thick split skin grafts of various sizes, and now we have electric dermatomes. In the early 1940's doctors were beginning to use homogenous grafts, from relatives or cadavers. These proved impermanent and gave way to autogenous grafts taken from the patient's own body.

For physicians and surgeons alike, the years immediately preceding World War II were a challenging time. The air was alive with exciting developments. And there were more to come.

VIII. War and Post-War Breakthroughs

The outbreak of World War II in 1939 brought the depression in Canada to an official end and in the field of medicine hastened the practical application of scientific developments in a number of important fields. Research that had been going on for years suddenly came out into the open and products became available that affected family medicine all over the world.

I can never forget the fall months of the later 1930's and early 1940's, when polio annually was casting a chill of fear over Lucknow district people. The late summer months of 1937 and 1941 were particularly bad ones with the disease causing the deaths of a score or more of our young people.

There were two young women with chest muscle paralysis so severe they required hospital treatment in iron lungs. One, from a family with three polio victims, was rushed to London Hospital in September 1937 to be put into an iron lung. She was seventeen and recovered, to live for ten years or so with the occasional aid of a respirator, but her nineteen-year-old brother, admitted to the hospital a few days after she was, died within a couple of days. His illness was diagnosed as poliomyelitis. On the day of his funeral, another brother of nine entered the hospital with a mild attack of the same disease—and recovered.

In another family, a father and son were afflicted at the same time and, strangely enough, each was left with the same muscle weakness, that of the left upper arm.

No wonder the citizens were in a near-panic. It was a terrifying experience for me during one of these epidemics to watch my two youngest children, Nancy two and Bruce eight, lie ill for two days with a fever, headache and stiff neck, wondering helplessly when paralysis would appear as it had with so many neighbors. I even briefly questioned my wisdom in staying with my community rather than fleeing with the family to a non-epidemic district.

My fears and frustrations probably were not unlike those of people during the plagues of Europe during the Middle Ages. It has been estimated that the Black Death in the 14th Century killed forty-three million persons. In France and Italy it wiped out half their populations. For lack of burial ground, rivers—after being blessed by the Pope—were turned into graveyards for thousands of victims. Another statistic according to the *Encyclopedia Britannica* is that during the Great Plague of London of 1664-65, Parliament met in Oxford while the King and Court fled the city with two-thirds of its inhabitants, the population then being estimated at 460,000. The people of that day knew that bubonic plague, typhus, smallpox, cholera, etc., were contagious and believed they were transmitted by some sort of poison in the air. The only defense they knew was to put the greatest possible distance between themselves and the sick. Even a few doctors ran away.

Lucknow people in 1937 knew that medical authorities believed poliomyelitis to be due to a virus—an agent so small it hadn't yet been seen through a microscope—and they suspected it was spread by house flies carrying the virus from the feces of patients. If this was true, where could they be safe? In August and September the flies were swarming in all houses, and a great number of them had only outdoor toilets.

The incidence of polio in Ontario for the years 1920-1969 from the annual reports of the Ontario Department of Health, not including deaths, is charted:

1920 – 37	1925 – 92	1930 – 471	1935 – 108	1940 – 87
1921 – 81	1926 – 271	1931 – 161	1936 – 208	1941 – 140
1922 – 205	1927 – 51	1932 – 175	1937 – 2,544	1942 – 89
1923 – 19	1928 – 85	1933 – 53	1938 – 160	1943 – 81
1924 – 84	1929 – 477	1934 – 326	1939 – 216	1944 – 333

1945 – 143	1950 – 372	1955 – 169	1960 – 45	1965 – —
1946 – 512	1951 – 1,699	1956 – 193	1961 – 23	1966 – —
1947 – 792	1952 – 699	1957 – 65	1962 – 19	1967 – —
1948 – 370	1953 – 2,109	1958 – 20	1963 – —	1968 – —
1949 – 1,235	1954 – 250	1959 – 228	1964 – 2	1969 – 2

These incidence statistics show: 1) that of the two severe local epidemics of 1937 and 1941, only 1937 appears to have been part of a province-wide visitation; 2) that 1957 ushered in a permanent annual decrease in the number of cases, due to Salk vaccine, which was first introduced for general use by the Connaught Medical Research Laboratories in 1955; 3) that polio began to disappear completely in Ontario during some years beginning with 1963. This is in marked contrast to Mexico where it was still a serious disease in the late 1960's.

In 1941 I called upon the provincial Department of Health for counsel and help. One of its research workers looked the situation over and gave it as his opinion that the outbreak, though particularly severe, was local. Probably all the village children had had the infection, he suggested, and by way of proving this he asked for specimens of feces from as many children as possible who were healthy and had not been ill all summer. The idea was to inject extracts of the specimens into Rhesus monkeys and wait one to three weeks to see if they developed polio. This was the only reliable way of testing for the virus, though it was expensive as the monkeys cost $25.00 each. I was able to send him feces specimens from thirty-two children whose parents assured me they had not been ill for many months. The researcher put the thirty-two specimens into six groups and injected their abstracts into as many monkeys, later reporting that five developed poliomyelitis.

Infection with the polio virus causes a wide range of illness symptoms, but every infection from mild to severe confers a permanent immunity on the individual; never again need he fear having the disease.

Of the many kinds of polio there were dozens and dozens of the *mild-non-paralytic* type. Probably four to five per cent of those infected in the days before vaccination had a non-paralyzing illness. These were of two grades: a) the mildest of all, with a low fever, like that of a cold, with weakness and loss of appetite and lasting only a couple of days; b) the same symptoms as "a" to which was added some stiffness and soreness of the posterior muscles of the neck. Usually this too lasted only two or three days though I recall a girl of five lying for a week with a fever and stiff neck. I always considered the presence of a stiff neck, along with a fever and perhaps headache, proof positive of a polio infection.

The *paralyzing type of polio* was the one that spread such a pall of alarm and gloom over our community. Probably one to two per cent of infected persons suffered a measure of nerve damage, ranging in severity from some limited muscle paralysis to a fatal outcome. This type also was of two grades:

a) The spinal form was characterized by weakness of the muscles of the neck, abdomen, trunk, diaphragm, chest or limbs. Sudden paralysis of legs in a youth is a shattering experience. One young man of twenty, paralyzed to the waist, wept uncontrollably at the slightest reference to his illness. Visitors were cautioned to avoid any reference whatever to it. This was in marked contrast to Lorne, a boy in the country who was stricken in his mid-teens. For two days it was only a mild fever and stiff neck. On the third day, weakness of his feet appeared. Each succeeding day examination showed a steady extension of the weakness upward. This ascending paralysis didn't stop until his legs were completely useless. In treatment he persisted faithfully in trying to make them useful again. He obtained a wheelchair, left his farm home to learn the trade of a shoemaker, and is now a self-supporting citizen. Though he had a lot of medical care, including periods of therapy in London and Toronto hospitals, the chief factor in his rehabilitation was his unfailing cheerfulness and his determination never to give up.

b) The *bulbar form* of the paralyzing type of polio was a particularly dangerous condition where the virus invaded the basal part of the brain which houses the vital centers controlling our breathing and heart action. I lost two patients with this type within two weeks, both boys in their late teens. They died suddenly without warning, just appeared to stop breathing. Had I been with them at the time I would have tried artificial respiration. A third similar fatality seemed to be impending. A neighbor, a sixteen-year-old boy, after two days of the mild polio illness, suddenly became worse with fast unsteady breathing, a fast irregular pulse and a little trouble in swallowing. I phoned Toronto for a consultant. He arrived, and on our way to see the patient he remarked casually, "I have never seen one of these bulbar types." This shocked me. There had evidently been some misunderstanding about the type of aid I wanted. I might need someone to put a breathing tube into the patient's trachea. I stayed with the boy all night because I wanted to try artificial respiration if he stopped breathing. In my office I had a small aspirator set up to take over and suck phlegm from his throat if needed. It wasn't needed, however. He lived through the night, recovered and was left with only wasting of the muscles of his left shoulder and arm.

There was some doubt in those days about the best early treatment of muscle weakness. Medical advice was to put the paralyzed limbs to rest in proper position with light plaster-of-paris splints and later start massage and encourage movement. Then Sister Kenny in the United States, with much fanfare, advised hot packs and massage early. Though this didn't do all she said it would, she made a valuable contribution in the early use of heat and massage, which was soon recognized as preferable to splinting.

Amid the uncertainties in our knowledge of polio, in one epidemic year of the early 1940's medical authorities suggested we might prevent infection by spraying the posterior nasal passages and upper throat of children with a solution of zinc sulphate. We did this to hundreds of children in the office that fall. It must have been unsuccessful, as we didn't repeat it the next year.

I referred earlier to a researcher from the provincial Department of Health who tested feces samples to show that many of our village children during an epidemic had had the infection. This research worker in 1941 wanted to test a couple of other ideas. He asked for flies to be collected from a house where there was a child ill with polio. I had one in mind, a house a mile in the country swarming with flies where a girl of five lay ill for ten days with a fever and stiff neck. Her two younger sisters filled a one-ounce bottle with house flies which I gave to the researcher, who in turn refrigerated them until the following winter. At that time he tested them on a monkey for polio virus and reported that they carried a virulent strain.*

He wondered also if any of the recovered polio victims were still harboring the virus a year later. I was able to send him feces specimens from six recovered patients a year after they had been ill. He reported finding virus in one specimen.

I have hesitated to report these findings of the research worker as I do not have his permission, nor do I remember his name. I am aware that it is his privilege to report on the work he did. However, I do not think the findings were orginal discoveries; I believe he was trying to prove the findings of other researchers.

A word about viruses, which are a group of minute infectious agents. Some infect plants, others cause animal diseases, and some even attack bacteria. The polio virus is one of the smallest of those attacking animals. *The Oxford Dictionary* defines a virus as a poison of contagious disease, and the word was applied first by Pasteur to the invisible infective agent of rabies. Viruses are smaller entities than germs or bacteria and quite different, appearing to be more primitive in that they are living creatures which can change into non-living matter. For instance, they can crystallize and in the crystal form are as inert as grains of sand. In a proper environment where temperature and moisture are favorable, however, these crystals can blossom forth into life

* Today's authorities agree that the polio virus infests the gastro-intestinal tract of the victim and that flies can carry it to others in an epidemic, but they are not sure this is the usual mode of spread.

again, grow, multiply, and destroy the living cells of the host plant or animal.

One of these small virus agents has recently been identified and given the name Virus (T1). It is very vicious, lives only on bacteria or germs, and its favorite host is *Escherichia coli*—a species of organisms constituting the greater part of the intestinal flora of man and animals. The virus is so virulent that when it enters a bacteria cell it immediately destroys the cell's nucleus and can produce one hundred progeny within thirteen minutes.

These agents are measured in microns; a micron is a millionth of a meter and a meter is 39 1/3 inches long. T1 is 150 millimicrons long and its head 50 millimicrons, which means it must be magnified one hundred thousand times for the researcher to see it. That he can see it is due to the electron microscope developed in 1937 which came into general use in the 1960's.

We now have two excellent vaccines for the control of paralytic poliomyelitis:* first, the injectable Salk vaccine and, second, the oral Sabin vaccine. Their development makes an exciting success story, partly because our knowledge of the virus itself is scant, but more so because brilliant cooperative planning brought them forth. Furthermore, their production demonstrates superbly how many serious diseases have been mastered by prevention rather than by treatment measures.

An early event of primary importance was the establishment in 1938, through the efforts of Franklin D. Roosevelt, of the National Foundation for Infantile Paralysis (NFIP). From this date onward most of the research on poliomyelitis in America was stimulated and financed by the NFIP, which raised its funds by public subscription.

After the Second World War breakthroughs began to come. By 1949 three major types of polio virus were identified and numbered: Types I, II and III. They were not all of the same virulence. This discovery showed some of the extent of the problem. Then it was discovered that the virus could be grown

* Dr. J. K. W. Ferguson, Director, Connaught Medical Research Laboratories, Toronto. (Extract from brochure.)

on monkey kidney tissue. Up to then it was thought to grow only on human nervous tissue cells. Finally, workers at the Connaught Medical Research Laboratories in Toronto in 1949 produced a solution called Medium 199 in which cells in tissue culture with the polio virus would grow and thrive.

With these tools at hand, Dr. Jonas Salk in Pittsburgh in 1950 undertook to produce and test a vaccine on a small scale. The Connaught Laboratory workers went ahead and, on invitation of the NFIP, produced more than three thousand litres of tested virus of all types which was inactivated in the United States. By this we mean that its potency was weakened down by formalin until it would not cause paralytic polio on injection into humans. They were now ready in 1954 for a trial of unprecedented magnitude.

A campaign was organized to inject two million children, most of them in forty-four States of the United States, but some in Finland and some in two Canadian provinces. They used a poly virus, that is a mixture of the three major types. Some children were given injections of the vaccine, a second group were given a harmless injection of similar appearance, namely 199. Neither the children, parents nor doctors giving the injections knew who received the vaccine and who did not, until the results were collected and analyzed. A third group of children selected as similar in age, sex and social circumstances were given nothing but were kept under medical supervision for six months.

This was the most ambitious public health research or field testing ever attempted. It cost $7,500,000, and the whole research program going back to 1938, over thirty million.

Then in May 1955 tragedy struck in the United States and almost ruined the future of Salk vaccine. Cases of paralytic poliomyelitis broke out following injections until they numbered seventy-nine. The vaccination program was halted. When the investigation was completed, it was apparent that nearly all the polio cases were associated with a few lots of vaccine from one manufacturer. In Canada half a million doses of vaccine had been given without any paralytic polio appearing, so the Canadian authorities continued their program until two million children were vaccinated—and there was still no trouble. The United States health authorities were encouraged by Canadian action and resumed production of the vaccine with new regulations for manufacturing and testing which were so stringent it is astounding that any vaccine was ultimately released.

In spite of many difficulties the provincial departments of health across Canada, after exhaustive tests and widespread observations, have indicated that Salk vaccine in Canada has been at least 90 to 95 per cent effective.

The alternative to injectable Salk vaccine now available is live polio virus vaccine for oral use, or more briefly Sabin vaccine, to name it for its inventer and sponsor, Dr. Albert Sabin of Cincinnati.

At about the time that Dr. Salk began the development of a killed injectable poliomyelitis vaccine, three investigators—including Dr. Sabin—began each independently to develop a live vaccine that could be taken by mouth. The advantages of an oral vaccine are three: it eliminates injections, it is more economical as less vaccine is needed per dose, and with its use a more rapid control of epidemics is possible.

Dr. Sabin's oral vaccine gained acceptance largely as a result of tests on monkeys, but partly because it had been accepted by the country of his birth, Russia, and given there to millions of children with no apparent harm. In 1962 it was accepted in Canada, and millions of doses of trivalent Sabin vaccine have been made and distributed by Connaught Laboratories to countries around the world, to be used without mishap.

Both the Salk and the Sabin vaccines are so safe and effective it is sometimes hard to know how best to use our wealth of resources. The risks from their use must be extremely small. For the time being the United States and most Canadian provinces use the Sabin oral vaccine as the one of choice in community programs. The Salk vaccine seems to be the choice for routine immunization, especially for infants and children. The details of the use of the vaccines vary somewhat from province to province in Canada.

In Ontario various combinations of Salk vaccine with other antigens are available and effective. For instance, there is a combination of tetanus toxoid and Salk vaccine. Also a combination of diphtheria toxoid, tetanus toxoid, whooping cough vaccine and Salk vaccine.

Polio with its chill of fear is past. In fact, with our vaccines polio now is a forgotten disease.

While early research leading to the polio vaccines was going on, and yearly outbreaks of the disease were stressing the urgency of that problem, there were other important developments in the field of antibiotic medicine. Some of it was the culmination of research done nearly two decades before.

Liver therapy had radically altered the treatment for pernicious anemia in the 1920's, but it was not until the mid-forties that a group of chemists finally succeeded in isolating the anti-pernicious factor in liver and obtained the beautiful red crystals of a compound known now as Vitamin B_{12}. Though there are still some unanswered questions about its use, it is unique in that it contains cobalt and it has proved to be a convenient and inexpensive therapy superior to liver and a marvellous aid in diagnosing and controlling the disease. Today it is possible to diagnose a case of anemia through estimation of Vitamin B_{12} in the blood after treatment has been suspended for six months. Also, a specific diagnosis is now available by a study of the bone marrow. So effective is the modern treatment that the life-expectancy of patients suffering from anemia has been increased by many years. One patient I know of is quite well after forty-three years of liver and Vitamin B_{12}. But though the advances have been spectacular, some mystery still remains. Occasional patients will have advanced nervous system changes with little blood change, while others will have the typical blood picture and little neurological change. There is no agreement yet on the optimum maintenance dose of Vitamin B_{12}. Curiously, for some unknown reason, there are today fewer pernicious anemia patients in certain areas of the world, such as Toronto and New York, while it remains a common illness in the Maritimes, the British Isles and the Scandinavian countries.

The search for the best cure goes on and researchers are still from time to time stumbling up blind alleys.

The mass production of penicillin in 1945 was perhaps the most spectacular breakthrough of the decade. As noted in Chapter III, Sir Alexander Fleming of St. Mary's Hospital in London, England, had observed a mold on a culture plate that apparently destroyed staphylococcus germs and in 1928 named the unknown substance penicillin, suggesting that it might be useful in treating infections. The suggestion was ignored until World War II when England was fighting for survival and had a desperate need for better treatment of military and civilian infectious casualties.

A group of researchers at Oxford University undertook to isolate enough penicillin to test on a patient and extracted a few grains of a yellowish-brown powder. The first therapeutic injection was given in February 1941 to a London policeman who was near death from an infection. He rallied and seemed on the road to recovery, but as there was no more penicillin, he died.

Small supplies of this wonder drug were built up with difficulty. Most of the first half-dozen patients were youngsters because their small body size required only small doses. In a desperate effort to extend the supply, penicillin was extracted from the patient's urine for re-use. All evidence indicated that it was a life-saving substance of unimaginable potency, but it was needed by the ton instead of the grain. Then, in 1945 mass production was achieved in the United States.

With this new addition to the arsenal of drugs, the antibiotic epoch which began in the 1930's with sulfanilamide and its successors was proceeding apace. It ushered in wonderful changes. For instance, as late as 1919 Sir William Osler, the dean of Canadian physicians, recommended blood-letting in the treatment of pneumonia. In the mid-twenties in large general hospitals in Canada the death rate from that disease was 20 to 30 per cent. Now recent statistics show that in the same hospitals, with the aid of penicillin, it has shrunk to 3 to 5 per cent. No longer does the patient have to pay for tanks of oxygen, days of twenty-four-hour nursing care and long hours of a doctor's time. Many suffering from the disease no longer even need to be hospitalized as the infection can be stopped abruptly at home in the early stages.

Tubercular patients were to share in the benefits of medical discoveries during the mid- and late forties.

Tuberculosis, long a mysterious disease, had been studied for many years with substantial gains in understanding its nature. Surgeons especially were doing very useful work in controlling it during the first quarter of the century (see Chapter III) and its highly infectious character was recognized by 1937 when the pasteurization of all milk sold in Ontario became compulsory. In 1940 research was intensified by the start of Christmas Seal campaigns to raise money for films and clinics.

After that chemotherapy with its wonder drugs for the tubercular brought about what seemed to be overnight changes. Streptomycin and para-amino-salicylic acid (PAS), a cousin of aspirin, came into use in 1948, to be followed by the discovery of isoniazid in 1952. These drugs in various combinations proved amazingly successful in destroying the tubercle bacillus germ. *Intensive therapy with these drugs could stop the cough of a patient within twenty-four hours.* And stopping the cough, it was learned, was the chief aid in finally gaining a large measure of control over the spread of the disease. The new drugs did it.

Isoniazid was synthesized in 1912 at the time Ehrlich discovered an arsenic compound in the treatment of syphilis. It was first used in 1952 in the treatment of T.B. patients in a Staten Island sanatorium. Combined with streptomycin and

PAS it was found to weaken the resistance of the tubercle bacilli to these antibiotics.

It is believed that about 7 per cent of people exposed to tubercular infection will develop the disease, i.e., the morbidity rate is said to be about 7 per cent. The surgeons of pre-drug days had already come to appreciate the importance of eliminating the patient's cough as a means of controlling the disease—by putting the diseased lung at rest they helped reduce the coughing. In the early days of chemotherapy there was a marked upsurge of thoracic surgery because the patients became safer risks, but as time went on doctors began giving antibiotics for longer periods with a view to eliminating surgery altogether. Now there is little thoracic surgery; phrenic nerve crushes and thoracoplasty are eliminated and pneumothorax remains only as a continuation of past treatment.

The total picture today is very different from what it was. There is now a higher percentage of older people with tuberculosis. There is at present a small percentage of children, and this was true in the 1920's because tuberculosis of the lung is not primarily a children's disease. But children can become susceptible and later on develop the adult type of infection. Today the search for victims of the disease takes more effective forms than in the past. There are now industrial and community surveys, chest X-rays of patients admitted to general hospitals, and clinics for detection working in places like jails and mental hospitals where there is a high incidence of the disease. (Tubercular surveys of the mentally ill started in 1929 and surprised everyone by revealing a considerably higher incidence of the disease than among the general population.) With the advent of the new drugs, too, the period of treatment was drastically shortened: a stay of three months in hospital now is average for minimal cases, six for moderately advanced cases and nine for the far advanced. Treatment in sanatoria is free, drugs are free to patients at recognized chest clinics and from physicians specializing in the chest. As a result, in short, there is now not much tuberculosis—it belongs to a vanishing age.

Another illness of the lungs that yielded to wonder drugs was the dread disease of bronchiectasis, where the lung is really rotting away with multiple small abscesses. These patients are marked by extreme pallor, an incessant cough and fetid sputum, and the only known relief in the 1920's was achieved by removal of the diseased part. Today, with the help of wonder-drug antibiotics and postural drainage, bronchiectasis has become a medical rather than surgical problem, and the life-expectancy now of a patient is only about three years short of normal. Thirty years and more ago few lived past their fortieth year. The fearsome ailment of lung abscess was unyielding to treatment until the breakthrough with sulfa drugs.

Although that old common misery, the head cold, is still with us, its characteristics seem to have altered during the last thirty years. In the past we saw many sufferers with their whole nasopharynx stuffed up with a profuse nasal discharge, and sometimes there was an accompanying earache. Today the head cold still involves the nasal passages but its chief features are often an upper respiratory or chest infection with a sore throat, much coughing, perhaps a mild fever and *much less nasal discharge*. I have no idea what has brought about this change in symptoms. Could it be that the widespread use of antibiotics has altered the nature of the pool of germs causing the old-style ailment? We know that other germs have been changed by their environment.

In the Trueman Wood Lecture delivered before the Royal Society of Arts in London, 1963, Professor Chain declared: "Drugs are one of our greatest blessings—perhaps the greatest—of our time." He went on to say that he could do without the means of fast locomotion which modern technology has made available to us, be it motor cars, trains or jets, and could live very nicely without a wireless or television set, in fact does, and could at a pinch even do very well without electric light—but he shudders at the thought of having to undergo the torture of the extraction of a wisdom tooth without a local anesthetic; and much worse still is the thought of having a limb amputated or an appendix removed without a general anesthetic.

Many people would say amen to this.

The following table taken from the Trueman Wood Lecture referred to above shows what a dramatic effect anti-bacterial agents have had on the mortality rate in our time:

DEATH RATE 1920-1960 FROM SELECTED CAUSES

Cause of Death	*Death Rate per 100,000 Population*				
	1920	*1930*	*1940*	*1950*	*1960*
Tuberculosis, all forms	113.1	71.1	45.9	22.5	5.9
Dysentery, all forms	4.0	2.8	1.9	0.6	0.2
Diphtheria	15.3	4.9	1.1	0.3	0.0*
Whooping cough	12.5	4.8	2.2	0.7	0.1
Meningococcal infections	1.6	3.6	0.5	0.6	0.3
Measles	8.8	3.2	0.5	0.3	0.2
Influenza and Pneumonia, except pneumonia of newborn	207.3	102.5	70.3	31.3	36.6
Gastritis, Duodenitis, Enteritis, Colitis	53.7	26.0	10.3	5.1	4.2
Deliveries and complications of pregnancy, childbirth and puerperium	19.0	12.7	6.7	2.0	0.8
Certain diseases of early infancy	69.2	49.6	39.2	40.5	37.0

* 1959 (figure for 1960 not available).

As a result of drug therapy and improved hygiene the average life expectation has been extended about ten years:

AVERAGE LIFE EXPECTATION

Year	*Number of Years*
1930	59.7
1940	62.9
1959	69.7

IX. Sexuality and Some Related Problems

Looking back, I am astonished how little sexuality was discussed by my patients. The Scots are a reticent and disciplined people, which may in part explain it. Also, the times were different, and the freedoms of speech and conduct being exercised in more worldly urban areas during and after the "roaring twenties" were perhaps slow in reaching us. However, the subject did crop up occasionally.

A Mrs. D. was in hospital where she had given birth to her fifth baby in five years. This was in the mid-1930's, about the time it was accepted that we could safely shorten the stay in bed after childbirth to six days instead of the traditional ten to fourteen days. On the fifth day I announced to my patient that she could go home the next morning. When I returned the following day she was in tears.

"Please, may I stay a couple more days?" she begged.

"Why do you ask?"

"I want another two days away from my husband. He has had intercourse every night since we were married."

"Why don't you say no sometimes?" I asked. It seemed to me a reasonable question.

"He would be angry. It is his right as a husband."

What a world of inner conflict and accommodation must have lain behind that statement!

And there was the other extreme. Sam and Mary (these are not real names) were married in their mid-thirties. Ten years later Sam casually informed me that they had never consummated their marriage. I didn't credit him with that much moderation, so I didn't quite believe him. However, I had to change my opinion some years after that, when Mary was in hospital and I had occasion to verify the fact that she was still a virgin.

Sexual problems take an infinite variety of forms, and each individual has his or her own way of dealing with them. It was in the spring that the mother of several fine children came to see me from a neighboring town. She was a forceful, aggressive type; later I learned that she was the driving force behind the successful business she and her husband managed.

"Doctor, I wish to ask an unusual question," she began. "My husband places so much importance on sex it disgusts me. He will spend many hours of a night in sexual activity. My question is—are all men like this?"

"My dear lady," I replied, "I am not an authority on how men behave in bed. I'm not sure, but I believe most men are not like your husband."

"I will find out. I'm taking the children away for the summer. I may be back in six months or I may never come back."

"If you return," I suggested, "please come in and tell me about yourself."

Six months later she appeared in the office with this story:

"I lived for periods of one month each with two men. I know now that many other men are not like my husband. But now I am pregnant. Will you look after me?"

I said that I would. "But what will your husband say about this?"

"I have enough on him to make him behave. For years he has left at intervals of six weeks or more, with no word of where. I know more than he thinks about these holidays. I can handle him."

The pregnancy proceeded normally and everything appeared serene on the home front.

There stays in my mind the remark of one of our married leading citizens who confided to me that he was not interested in sexual intercourse; it was such a vulgar form of activity. His wife probably taught him this.

The problem of incest I encountered only once, and then only as a probability. Two unmarried sisters became pregnant at a one-year interval. They weren't very bright, but bright enough to refuse to tell either me or the Children's Aid Society the name of the man responsible. There was some evidence that it was incest with their father the culprit. When this sort of thing happened in ancient Greece the mother and children sometimes killed the father—blood revenge. However, in this instance the girls took their babies home to care for them and all remained peaceful.

It has been suggested that in a community of Scotch Presbyterians there would not be much venereal disease, meaning gonorrhea and syphilis—or the twin sisters, as they are occasionally called. This is to infer that the canny Scots are too close-fisted to frequent brothels. It is a slightly erroneous supposition. Lucknow district did not have a great incidence of the disease but it had its share. In the 1920's and '30's I was seeing at least six to eight patients a year with acute gonorrhea, and all but one of them were men. Few women consulted me with symptoms suggestive of gonococcal infection. The only one I recognized had a severe infection complicated by the possibility of acute appendicitis. She was so seriously injured by the disease she could never have a baby—which was not surprising as sterility in such instances was common in women. As for syphilis, I saw about ten patients in two decades. However, these afflicted people presented more interesting and unusual features than their mere numbers suggest.

For a long time these quite different infections were considered to be the same. As late as the 18th century, the famous Dr. John Hunter attempted to determine whether gonorrhea was distinct from syphilis by inoculating himself with pus from a patient supposedly ill with gonorrhea, and a typical sore of syphilis developed. From this he concluded the diseases were one and the same, and this was believed until a doctor by the name of Record later established the identity of each.

Gonorrhea is the earliest recorded disease of man. It is a specific infection of the urethra and other passages due to a germ called gonococcus. Hippocrates thought it was due to overactivity of the gonads, which explains its name (gonus = semen + rhoi = a flow). Mosaic laws in The Book of Leviticus, Chapter XV, verses 2-11, refer to it as a "running issue of the flesh," the Hebrew word for penis being the same as for flesh.

The amours of Casanova (*circa* 1760) were interrupted by a number of attacks of gonorrhea, for which he treated himself very intelligently: he kept away from physicians whose treatment he despised; he went to bed for six weeks and took a light diet. At the end of this time he seemed to be quite well again.

As a rule the disease is transmitted by sexual intercourse, commonly illicit, although there are always some patients who suggest otherwise. "Doctor, could I have got this off a toilet seat?" is one familiar question. And there are the bashful young men who announce to the doctor that they have "contracted a cold." In one such instance a doctor I heard of, knowing the jargon, said, "Let me see it," and after gazing upon the offending organ, which had all the clinical signs and symptoms of an acute urethral discharge, said, "Man, until that either coughs or sneezes, I'd call it clap."

Annually in the 1930's there were about one million cases of acute gonorrhea in the United States and Canada, in addition to another million requiring treatment for the disease's ravages. It was much more prevalent than any other communicable illness, and nearly half of those suffering from it acquired the infection before the age of twenty-five.

After an incubation period of three or four days, or a little longer, the patient notices a urethral discharge. There may be so much local pain that it is difficult for the patient to move about, or the degree of discomfort may be minor. Local complications may develop, especially if the infection travels upward in the urethra which it usually does.

The approved treatment before modern drugs were available was to irrigate or wash out the urethra and bladder with a warm solution of 1-in-5,000 potassium permanganate. A large enema can to hold this solution was hung on the wall near the office toilet. A rubber tube led from the bottom of the container to which could be attached a catheter with an irrigating tip. The patient was told to insert the catheter into the urethra and up into the bladder by attempting to relax the bladder sphincter voluntarily. If the solution washed out the bladder, he was considered to have had a good irrigation. The patient would come in every day or so and give himself a bladder lavage. It was a painful procedure, but no more so than the disease. One could hear the patient grinding his teeth and swearing to himself as he went about his task.

This treatment was taught at medical school and was popular in large city hospitals, though it was not as good therapy as that of Casanova. If the patient did not have a higher-up infection, such as a posterior urethritis, when he first came in he surely had one after a few days of bladder irrigations, because one thing we accomplished was to wash the germs higher up. It required six weeks or so of irrigations for the acute condition to subside.

There were other treatments. Sometimes we injected 20 per cent Argyrol into the urethra or Neo-Silvol, a silver protein product. For instance, Argyrol drops for use in the eyes could prevent a gonorrheal opthalmia, a serious infection when it occurred; fortunately I never saw it.

The varied types of this disease are best illustrated by some of my patients.

William Mac (not his real name), a six-foot two-hundred-pound Scotsman, consulted me for a urethral discharge.

"Do you know what this is?" I asked him.

"Yes, I do."

"Where did you get it?"

"I was west on the Harvesters' Excursion and on the way home I stopped for a night in Regina."

This was in the late twenties when hundreds of men from Ontario went west yearly, for a railway return fare of twenty dollars, to help farmers harvest their wheat.

William Mac was put on the usual bladder-irrigation treatment. In a few days he was worse, being more feverish and toxic, and was told to stay in bed. I would visit him regularly and I left with him antiseptic bichloride tablets for making solutions with which to wash his hands, face and genitals at frequent intervals. He was warned that the tablets were highly poisonous.

A couple of days later his mother called frantically to say her son had swallowed two of the poisonous tablets. I went out at once as they were enough to kill him. As I rapidly prepared to wash out his stomach he confessed, "Doctor, at the last minute I lost my nerve. They are under my pillow."

This alerted me to what a sensitive man he was and what might happen and did happen to him. He was sure he would not recover from the infection, and "would never be clean again." Like many seriously ill people he had to be told repeatedly that he *would* recover, but this wasn't enough. He became mentally unbalanced and was referred to a consultant in London who had him confined for ten days or so in an Ontario mental hospital, followed by a few days in a general hospital to clear up an abscess.

The most encouraging thing about gonorrhea was that the patients rarely died of it. William finally recovered, being left with a urethral stricture which responded well to dilatation once a year with a set of urethral dilators.

At about the same time Tom, a big Irishman, consulted me with a complaint similar to William Mac's. Our interview followed much the same pattern:

"Where have you been?"

"I was on the Harvesters' Excursion and stopped over for a night in the city of Regina on the way home."

Tom too was put through the painful routine of bladder irrigations. I even showed more zeal with him as I added for good measure urethral injections of Neo-Silvol, the silver protein product. His progress followed the usual course. He began to improve in two or three weeks and recovered in six or eight weeks, the same length of time Casanova required for recovery.

While this case was in progress Ernest, another Scotsman, came in and casually asked if his slight discharge was serious. He had had it two weeks and it hadn't bothered him much.

"Where did you get this?"

"I was on the Harvesters' Excursion and stopped over for a night in Regina on the way back."

My smile must have given me away as he promptly asked, "Have others been in to see you?"

"Yes, two of them have. There are just two questions I wish to ask you: first, was the same woman with each of you?"

"Yes, she was."

"William has been very ill," I told him, "Tom is serious enough and you have such a mild case you can forget about it and go home, providing you don't do much work or drink any alcohol. My second question is: Can I guess the order of your procedure with this woman?"

"Yes, you can. It was one, two and three, as you have indicated."

In 1936, with the discovery of sulfanilamide, gonorrhea therapy changed radically. My friend, the late Dr. Jake Markowitz, a Toronto general practitioner, recalled how he tried some sample tablets on a bank teller and in three days wondered what had happened, the man seemed so well. This early wonder drug ushered in a new era for these patients. All we had to do was to give 80 grains for two days, 60 for two days, 40 for two days and 30 for two days, then 20 grains a day indefinitely. The cure was dramatic and seemed to be permanent. This treatment was later improved upon when penicillin became available in 1945.

Syphilis, gonorrhea's twin sister, is an infectious disease caused by a spirochete and usually transmitted by sexual contact.

There are two schools of thought with reference to the history of syphilis: the first holds that it has been in Europe from time immemorial; the second, that it was brought to Barcelona, Spain, from Haiti by the sailors of Christopher Columbus' fleet and that the army of Charles VIII in 1493 proceeded to syphilize Naples. Soon all Europe was infected. Paris reported in 1494 that the disease first became noticeably prevalent.

Syphilis was much more acutely serious in Columbus' day

than it is now. Benvenuto Cellini, the master goldsmith, in his autobiography at the age of fifty-eight, in 1559, said he suffered from it, and his monumental egotism and delusions of greatness possibly were due to its ravages.

The disease's violent secondary eruptions gave it the name of the "large pox," to differentiate it from the "small pox." The Shakespearian oath "a pox upon us" was the Elizabethan equivalent of "go to hell," or to the nether regions. Many early settlements in New England were founded largely to supply the London market with sassafras used as a remedy for various illnesses, chiefly syphilis.

In the early 1930's in the United States and Canada there were about 600,000 people with syphilis seeking medical care. About 70,000 children were born annually with it.

An elderly woman from a neighboring village consulted me about her husband of sixty-five. They had a family of seven children and he had been a successful merchant, but a change had come over him. His wife tearfully reported that she didn't think she could live with him much longer, he had grown so irascible and cantankerous—he even beat her at times. This was completely out of character and it was embarrassing to the family. On examining the man, I concluded that his altered behavior was probably due to senile changes. His blood tests proved normal, including that for syphilis. Six months later there was no improvement in his condition and, reviewing the whole problem of his difficult behavior for new clues, I drew off some spinal fluid for testing. It was reported positive for syphilis.

Finding this mature man with a form of brain syphilis surprised and confused me. He must have had the disease in his youth while living as a Cockney in London, England, though he denied all knowledge of any illness at that time. Here he was now with a wife and large family, all free of the disease, and he had shown no effects until the age of sixty-five.

In my days at medical school we were taught that syphilis was invariably a maimer or killer of mankind if untreated. No one ever suggested that people could recover from it unaided, and no one having it was advised to marry until after two years of therapy. Faced with this baffling case, I looked into the literature published on the subject since my graduation in 1923 and came upon interesting new findings. One report told of a Dr. Bruusgaard of an Oslo clinic who had followed 459 syphilitics for 15 years. After no treatment, or at best a little iodine and/or mercury by mouth, 25 per cent had a spontaneous cure and 64 per cent appeared to be individually unharmed. Of course, some of the latter would later show some of the disease's chronic effects.

I discovered also that in the 16th century Dr. Fracastorius wrote that he believed syphilis might die out of itself because it was so rapidly becoming milder. The truth is that the dreadful scourge had lost some of its virulence before the coming of modern medicine; the human race was developing an immunity to it. How had the medical profession forgotten what it really knew, namely, that there are always some human beings who prove resistant to new diseases? Nature has repeatedly demonstrated powers by which the race has survived a new disease eventually.

Shortly after syphilis appeared in Europe, mercury and guaiacum (a resin from certain tropical American trees) were introduced as remedies and later potassium iodine. They were responsible for some striking results. And in 1910, as I have said in an earlier chapter, the arsenical compound popularly called 606 was discovered, which destroyed the parasites without damaging the individual.

Armed with these assorted facts, some of them new to me, I treated my patient with an arsenical preparation and bismuth, which had replaced the earlier mercury. His fractious conduct was markedly modified, to the great relief of his family—though he lived only another two years.

In the 1940's I was pleased and maybe a little proud of the small blood-transfusion service I had organized for my patients. This was in the days before the Red Cross provided its magnificent service to hospitals. There were six young active and robust people on my list whose blood types I knew and whom

I could call upon when one of my patients needed blood. The local branch of the Red Cross paid the donor twenty-five dollars for each donation. I had no severe reactions with this service; the rubber-tubing equipment I was using was sterilized after each transfusion. I mention this because it was discovered in the mid-forties that most reactions were due to tiny particles of dried blood which had not been removed from the tubing—hence, today's use of plastic equipment.

Then my dream world of a satisfactory blood-transfusion service collapsed with a disastrous result for one patient. A middle-aged schoolteacher had a severe stomach hemorrhage and I called upon a young man from my small roster of donors with the appropriate blood type for a pint of blood. After cross-matching as a further check to see that there was no incompatibility, the patient was given the transfusion. Because of the distance to the hospital, I did this in the home with the help of my office nurse. This proved to be poor judgment because with the severe loss of blood it was particularly difficult to find a good arm vein, expose it and insert a cannula. However, the task was finally completed. The patient made splendid progress for some days, until a fever with a macular rash all over her body suddenly appeared. I had never seen anything like it and, on return to my office, it dawned on me that it might be syphilitic. To test this possibility, the woman was given penicillin which, in the presence of syphilitic infection, kills so many parasites at once that the patient has a very pronounced reaction with a high fever. Sure enough, two or three hours later she had a temperature of 106°. Her blood sample came back positive for this disease.

I hurried out to see the blood donor. He hadn't been ill. He hadn't been anywhere except around home—so he said. With his permission I took a blood sample, which was reported positive. Even in the face of this, he still continued quietly to deny any knowledge of any possible source of infection; he hadn't been to the city, etcetera. He added, "Perhaps I got it from a toilet seat, but if I have it, let's clear it up."

To say the least, it was shocking to ponder the fact that I, a physician, had given a patient this disease. It was a new twist in the practice of medicine. With visions of adverse publicity and a possible malpractice suit, I made a clean breast of the situation to my patient. Her answer was, "Don't worry, Doctor—you did the best you could and I am grateful for your help. No one but the three of us need to know anything about this." She was a forgiving soul if ever there was one!

This was in the early 1950's. Fortunately, penicillin had become available and it required only a few weeks to cure these two patients, as compared with a two-year regimen in the 1930's. Penicillin has, in fact, proved so effective in treating both gonorrhea and syphilis that—as someone has said—Sir Alexander Fleming "made lust safe for humanity." This is not precisely true because in the past few years gonorrhea has been increasing in Canada, and there is a resurgence of venereal disease in the United States.

This disaster to my patient was a further lesson to me. Obviously, doing blood tests on each of my donors every twelve months wasn't frequent enough. But fortunately the Canadian Red Cross had begun a national blood-transfusion service to supply every hospital in the country free of charge with whole blood, dried plasma, distilled water for its reconstitution and sterile administration sets, the one stipulation being that any hospital wishing to participate would make no charge whatsoever to the patients transfused under the plan. They opened their first depot in Vancouver in February 1947. The depot in London, from which my neighborhood hospital in Wingham was supplied, was set up in April 1959. Their plan covering all of Canada was in operation by 1961.

Following my unfortunate episode, I was delighted to give up my roster of blood donors in favor of the Red Cross service.

Another old recurring problem of sex is the unwanted pregnancy. The subject of abortion, so timely today, has always been controversial and full of complexities. I have been asked often: Who applied for abortions? and: Who were the abortionists?

These two questions always intrigued me. Though my experience with several score of abortions over the years probably doesn't qualify me as an authority, nevertheless I have been able to reach several personal conclusions.

Curiously perhaps, the single women asking for an abortion were greatly in the minority. Those I met were not feebleminded, notoriously promiscuous or from the wrong side of the street; most were bright intelligent girls. I would tell their mothers, "Don't throw in the sponge, after nine months of hell your daughter may make a wonderful woman." Many a woman needs a baby as a part of growing up—of becoming mature. One mother told me that early in life she decided she would contrive to have a baby whether married or not; she was going through life only once and wouldn't think of missing this experience. Having babies is a part of woman's normal functioning and not a disease.

Pregnancy for an unmarried girl is, of course, a tragedy. Possibly the only greater misfortune could be if twins were born. This happened to Jane Armour, Robert Burns' second wife, though in due course the children were legalized. None of the single unwed mothers I met repeated the experience. All of them were courageous and some incredibly so.

A young girl from Sault Ste. Marie came to visit her aunt and uncle in the country at Christmas. The day after her arrival she gave birth to a seven-month baby. It was probably the smallest infant I ever saw that lived; you could hold it in the palm of one hand. The mother took it to bed with her, where it thrived. Neighbors of the couple were told their niece was ill upstairs with a kidney infection and not once in the two weeks did the baby cry loud enough to be heard downstairs.

After the Christmas season the mother refused to consider parting with the child and took it home, prepared to be responsible for it on her meagre salary of a knitting factory employee. From Christmas greetings she sent me the next five years I knew that she continued to care for the child.

Single pregnant women in their dilemma frequently did bizarre things. One woman of twenty-five refused to marry the father when he proposed marriage after the birth. She no longer liked him because of his refusal of marriage before the event and chose the hard road of raising a daughter without a father. The child turned out to be a very fine girl indeed.

I remember making an initial visit to a woman of forty-five suffering from a persistent cough, to find her lying in a drafty upstairs bedroom in destitute surroundings, thin and terribly deformed with her knees drawn up nearly to her chin. She explained that she had been in bed nearly thirty years with arthritis. Though at first glance it looked like arthritis, I was sure after repeated examinations that it was not arthritis as we understand that disease. As I subsequently learned, her stay in bed dated from the birth of an illegitimate child in her late teens. She was so ashamed of having a child out of wedlock that she couldn't face her friends and neighbors, so just stayed in bed. Her type of leg contracture at the hips is a well-recognized form of deformity from long years of bed inactivity. She came by her strict moral code quite honestly; she was a Scotch Presbyterian of the old school.

Wisely, we were taught at medical school never to aid a woman to abort, and I learned early there must be no deviation from this policy. In trying to be kind and a little helpful to a woman pleading to be rid of her unwanted child, I told her there were no drugs known to be effective without poisoning her. As she was quite anemic, however, I suggested that perhaps some iron tablets would help restore her monthly periods if she was *not* pregnant. Unexpectedly and totally by coincidence, she had a miscarriage in a few days. Within a month no less than three women from different localities asked for tablets similar to those I gave Mrs. S. to bring on her abortion, and worst of all my confrère down the street intimated that I was acquiring a reputation for getting into the abortion business. This was a lesson to me. I must not give any impression whatever of aiding a pregnant woman to abort unless I was willing to become known as an abortionist—and quickly too.

As I have said, more married women than single asked for an abortion. The one most pronounced thing that characterized them all, married and single, was their coolly calculated willingness to resort to desperate measures even at the risk of their lives. Surely there must be a more humane and rational way for society to deal with this problem. But this is something else, which I will comment on later.

A farmer's wife, thirty years old, was pregnant for the third time. She had two robust sons in their teens at home and she didn't want another child. She was a healthy woman and there was no hint of marital trouble. In spite of my advice of caution, she insisted that she have an operation somewhere and if necessary would go to Detroit. I invited her to return to see me if she went through with her decision. She did, and came back with this story:

She had taken a morning bus to Detroit, a distance of a hundred and twenty-five miles down the Bluewater Highway. On arrival she went to a telephone booth, opened the directory at random and wrote down the names and addresses of doctors listed. The following morning she started to make the rounds. The first two doctors weren't interested. The third said, "My girl, I can't help you but my son down the hall may do so." He introduced her to his son who in a couple of days performed the operation in what she thought was his office. She returned home in a few days and at the time of our meeting was in good health.

Another farmer's wife with several children came in with the same request. On my refusal to assist, she declared her determination to interrupt the pregnancy and had already decided to call on a doctor some forty miles away who had a well-known reputation as an abortionist. So far as I knew, he was the only physician within a radius of a hundred miles who had this reputation. I had met him only once, at a county medical meeting, and remembered him as a saintly looking man of some seventy years with a heavily lined face and a magnificent shock of white hair.

My patient returned in a few weeks to tell me the outcome of the experience. The abortion had been performed, at a charge of $86.50—to be paid in advance. My guess is that $1.50 was for materials (probably laminaria stems) and $85.00 for the know-how. The woman was in difficulty, having only about half the fee with her, but the doctor accepted that and directed her to return for a second visit. On this occasion he demanded the rest of the fee. When she couldn't produce it he was very angry and became too familiar. My patient was a thrifty soul and loved a bargain and he probably guessed correctly that she really didn't intend to complete the payment so seized the opportunity for some illicit pleasure.

Every incident of abortion or attempted abortion had its own peculiar twist. An emergency call at daybreak of a beautiful June morning took me to a farm home seven miles into the country. The mother of two children was in shock for a miscarriage at seven months. She was as white as a sheet and gasping for breath at intervals. Her life was in danger from loss of blood. The nurse who accompanied me at once started intravenous fluids. (The introduction of quarts of intravenous glucose and saline solution was one of the most effective life-saving measures made available during my period of practice. I always had a supply in the office ready for any emergency.) Immediately we prepared to pack the woman's vagina, having brought along packing material, a speculum with its battery light and a long-handled forceps. (In case we were short of packing material, the nurse would sterilize a bed sheet by boiling in water and cut it into two-inch-wide strips. This careful and firm packing procedure would take about an hour and a half to complete. At the end of that time the bleeding would have ceased and the patient would be sitting up and asking for a drink—well on the road to recovery. The packing would be removed in about twelve hours.)

Though I had encountered several women in this dangerous condition, I was unable usually to learn whether the miscarriage was accidental or induced. The women wouldn't talk. This time I decided to see if I could find out what had started the difficulty. It looked suspiciously like deliberate interference by someone. As I made my way to the car, the husband following close behind, I suddenly turned to face him with the accusation: "You nearly killed your wife this morning. What did you do?"

This so surprised him, his lip dropped as he mumbled, "I used a catheter."

"Please let me see it."

He brought out a small rubber catheter—the common type.

"Who taught you how to use this?"

"Old Dr. . . . gave it to us many years ago and showed me how to use it."

Several years ago I had occasion to visit the Gatineau Memorial Hospital of Wakefield, Quebec, twenty miles or so from Ottawa. Here Dr. Harold Geggie, one of the grand old family doctors of Canada, and his three sons practiced group medicine in a clinic.

He showed me a five-day old baby with a three-inch long gash across its back over a shoulder blade. The history was that the mother had tried to bring on a miscarriage at seven and a half months by shooting herself in the abdomen with a "22." The bullet had gone in one side and out the other. She was sent into her local hospital in Hull, Quebec. Strange to say, nothing whatever happened and she went on to deliver herself at full term of this baby in the Wakefield hospital. There had been no healing whatever of the shoulder skin bullet wound while the baby was in the amniotic fluid of the womb. It was now healing nicely. (The Geggie's found nothing in the literature about the healing of intrauterine wounds. Later in the March 4, 1961 issue of the *Canadian Medical Association Journal*, Dr. Geggie's son, Dr. N. Stuart Geggie, reported this story and entitled it "Gunshot Wound of the Pregnant Uterus with Survival of the Fetus.")

One more example suggests the variety of the problems of the unwanted pregnancy. A schoolteacher from a neighboring town was five months pregnant at the age of forty-four. She was thoroughly disgusted with herself.

"You'd think a woman of my age would have enough sense not to get this way."

On my refusal to help, she gave me the name and address of a practical nurse in her town who performed such operations and who had promised to assist her. I heard no more from the teacher nor did I follow up on the volunteered information about the nurse abortionist, reasoning that the aim of medicine surely is not to reform people and make them virtuous; it is to safeguard their health and to rescue them from their vices and ailments.

From the evidence I think the reader may agree that the abortionists in my area were a motley group. Which is the only answer I can give to the question: Who were they?

Though the problem of abortions constituted a small part of my medical practice, I found it troublesome because it raised a number of health questions to which there are no easy answers. First, why should a pregnant woman who is determined not to have her baby be compelled to trust herself to a strange doctor, if she can find one willing to undertake the task—and, if not, to submit to incompetents working often under unsanitary conditions? Second, why do men have so much to say about abortions? Women have been having babies for a long time, and it is their bodies that are involved. Men's opinions about abortions seem often hollow and unrealistic. Surely they could put more trust in the judgment of women in a matter so close to them. Finally, "the opportunity to decide the number and spacing of children is a basic human right," as Secretary-General U Thant and many UN agencies have repeatedly said. If this is true, why doesn't society respect this right?

Roger Veylon* asserts that "woman is a superior creation biologically and the male just an addition to a basic feminine being. The Y chromosome is a degenerate X, which makes man a poor type of female. Boy meets girl in reproduction and girl does the rest. She can endure more, bear pain better and live longer, and from illness she bounces back faster. She is tougher mentally, far more males enter mental hospitals (in Canada at present only five per cent more), and more men commit suicide. Girls learn to read faster than boys and later on they make better drivers and have fewer fatal accidents."

* *Presse Med.* 79. 1587, 1967.

I don't know how much of this paragraph to believe, or I would be a member of Women's Lib.

I performed only one abortion. It was in the 1930's when an abortion in Ontario was legal if pregnancy endangered the life of the mother and if two doctors agreed to its interruption. In this instance it was done because of the mother's impaired heart. She was much sicker from the operation than I had expected, so sick that I vowed never to attempt another one. As the years went by, however, the possible conditions calling for abortion became fewer and fewer because we were steadily learning how to carry more and more pregnant women in poor health safely through childbirth.

All Catholic hospitals and some non-sectarian municipal ones in Ontario would not permit abortions. It took doctors many years to learn that the best treatment of a woman continuing to bleed after a miscarriage was to remove all womb contents by a so-called dilation and curettage. I remember performing such an operation on a very anemic woman whose fetus I was sure could not be living and being criticized sharply by a Catholic assistant superintendent of a non-sectarian hospital. The mother's health was much less important to her than was the baby, she told me. Of course, I thoroughly disliked sectarian medicine of this kind.

About 1965, in a special report based on a seven-year study of maternal deaths in Ontario, two leading obstetricians said there had been 35,000 abortions yearly in Toronto, compared with 42,000 live births in a population of nearly two million. Statistics show that there are probably 100,000 abortions annually in Canada, but this figure is only a shrewd guess as no one knows the precise number. The extent of the abortion problem would make a fruitful field of study for the College of Family Physicians. Family doctors with a little guidance could provide the answers.

The same obstetricians reporting above said abortion accounted for 69 out of 333 obstetrical deaths in Ontario between 1958 and 1963. Infection was the chief cause of death. About the same time the head of Metro Toronto Police Abortion Squad said that while most abortions were self-induced, some 5,500 a year were performed by abortionists for fees ranging from $150 to $1,500. Another statistic: in one year about ten abortionists were performing an average of one hundred operations per weekend.

Abortions are viewed differently in the various countries of the world and there is much disagreement. Powerful factions support arguments for and against the practice. As a result there is now an enormous literature on the subject.

The situation in the USSR interested me while I was there on a six-week visit in 1964. Makarov, a town some forty miles from Kiev, the capital of the Ukraine, has a district hospital serving an area with 100,000 people. In 1963 there were 1,900 live births and 1,200 abortions in this hospital. The birth rate in the USSR at the close of World War II was 23 per 1,000 population and this had fallen, as in the Makarov district, to 19 per 1,000 in 1963. Any woman in the USSR could have an abortion. Each of its large general hospitals had a doctor-lawyer official who dealt with abortions, divorces, changes in employment and even with the purchase of real estate. This official tried to discourage a woman from having an abortion, but he had no option but to grant it if she persisted. A recent regulation required that an abortion be entered on the woman's health card.

The superintendent of the Makarov hospital said there had been no mortality whatever from abortions performed in his hospital during the previous ten years. We expressed skepticism, as all surgical procedures have a mortality rate of some size. But he insisted his figures were correct. The same figures had been given the government, and if they were ever proved false he would lose his hospital-superintendent appointment. He justified the policy of doing all requested abortions in hospital by observing that if pregnant women don't want their babies they will find a dangerous way of dealing with them—and with this we certainly agreed.

I was told that not all members of the medical profession in the USSR were happy about the unlimited privilege given women to have abortions. Many doctors felt that perhaps it should be a one-performance privilege as the psychological effect on the mother is always quite profound. As a result of this professional uneasiness, a national committee was reviewing the situation. I do not yet know its conclusions.

I am now more inclined to believe the Makarov hospital's record of no maternal deaths from abortion in ten years. Recent figures from Hungary, Czechoslovakia and Jugoslavia, where legal abortions are performed freely, give their fatality rates as ranging from 3 to 5 per 100,000, which is very low indeed. By contrast, tonsillectomy cases in Canada produce 17 deaths per 100,000.

Most earlier societies, and many still today, neither prohibit abortion nor attach any stigma to it. For a long time our differing religious beliefs have influenced, rightly or wrongly, our thinking about it. Early Christian dogma, held that abortion is, like infanticide, murder, the killing of a human being—though the exact moment when the fetus acquires a rational soul and a life of its own has remained a matter of argument. The early Church set this point of "animation" at forty days after conception for a male child, eighty days for a female; abortions within that time limit were not a cause for excommunication, though still regarded as a serious sin. (English common law in the 18th century set the dividing line at the moment of "quickening," when the mother first felt the child stir in her womb—usually in the fifth month.) Then, in 1869 Pope Pius IX wiped out the forty-and-eighty-day rule and adopted the position that all abortions, at any period of fetal development, are murder, punishable by excommunication. This position is substantially unchanged by the pronouncement of the current Pope in 1971.

In practice, this means that if it comes to a choice between the life of the fetus and that of the mother, the fetus cannot be destroyed as a direct means of saving the mother's life. The natural death of mother and child, according to this view, is morally a lesser evil than the death of fetal life through abortion. Thus, today, no Catholic hospital or doctor may perform an abortion, even to save a mother's life.

Other religious positions on abortion are more lenient. The only policy statement from the combined Protestant churches in the United States is that made by the National Council of the Churches of Christ in 1961. Although stressing the sanctity of potential life, and condemning abortion as a method of family limitation, it approved legal hospital abortion "when the health or life of the mother is at stake." Inclusion of the crucial word "health" thus sets Protestant thinking far in advance of most laws.

Although Judaism has no central authority, in the Jewish tradition the embryo is not considered a living soul until its greatest part has emerged from the womb. Until that point, at least, the mother's life and health take precedence.

The situation in Ontario in regard to abortion has opened up greatly since the 1920's. Most accredited hospitals now have abortion committees of three or so doctors which assess and pass upon all abortion applications from their districts. They do not operate themselves. The conscience of the doctor who is authorized to do the abortion must be considered. If he doesn't want to perform it, he is under no obligation to do so. Also, the law has been liberalized. Abortion is now permissible if the health or life of the mother is endangered by continuance of the pregnancy. The significant word "health" has been added here and this is being interpreted quite broadly, with particular emphasis on the emotional effects on the mother.

Today, late pregnancies and many other undesired ones can be prevented by birth control pills and other contraceptive measures. Enovid, the first oral contraceptive, was marketed by G. D. Searle and Company in 1957. It was introduced as a therapeutic agent for painful menstruation, functional uterine bleeding, etc., but within a year its primary indication was changed to that of a contraceptive. Ortho-Novum was brought out in 1962 by Ortho Pharmaceutical (Canada) Ltd. This, as well as all future contraceptives, were introduced as such primarily, and secondly as therapeutic agents.

All oral contraceptives come from the *Dioscorea*, a genus of plants, the wild yams of Mexico, which grow abundantly in the state of Veracruz. It was in Veracruz Harbour, the most interesting way of entering the state even today, that Hernando Cortez landed his five hundred men in 1519 and immediately scuttled his ships to take his men on a seven-week march inland —beginning the destruction of the Aztec Empire of Montezuma II. It took many recent years of hard work and much brilliant research before the wild yams were tamed by chemists to yield a substance called *diosgenin*, the basic building block for the progestins, which in turn are combined with the female sex hormones like estrogen to form the oral contraceptives. Mexico now has a thirty-million-dollar-a-year yam industry, and so far this particular yam has refused to grow in any other country.

The subject of abortion is not in the main a happy one, so let me close on a cheerful note. Occasionally my advice not to interfere with a pregnancy was followed, as it was in the case of a mother of forty-five. She had raised four children—only the youngest, a girl of fourteen, remained at home—and she was greatly worried about having another child. She was sure her fourteen-year-old daughter would laugh at her as she wheeled a baby carriage down the street. In my time there was considerable support for this view. On screen, stage and TV the middle-aged woman who found herself pregnant was played for laughs. In real life, however, such an unwelcome fertility was often serious. The over-forty pregnancy with most of the children grown meant considerable disruption to a woman's life, and complications were likely if the woman suffered from diabetes, high blood pressure, arthritis or other ailments common to middle life. Also, mongoloid children are more frequently born to older women. In this instance, however, complications were not indicated and the woman was persuaded to go through with the pregnancy. I was rewarded several years later when she thanked me profusely for my advice. She and her husband had had more pleasure from this child than from any of the earlier ones.

X. Cancer: Hope Is a Sustaining Force

No affliction that man is heir to is quite so heavily weighted with dread and mystery as cancer. The word itself to many is synonymous with protracted suffering and death.

I found that cancer patients were worthy of special study. Standing out above all else was their loneliness and I tried to understand how men and women facing imminent dissolution alone saw the world, how they could overcome unimaginable difficulties to think and work when life was closing its doors. Like the Ancient Mariner:

> . . . this soul hath been
> Alone on a wide, wide sea:
> So lonely 'twas, that God Himself
> Scarce seemèd there to be.

In return for my efforts to understand, these patients taught me much. Through their loneliness could be heard their call for a measure of hope, a need to be treated as interesting persons and not shuffled into a corner to die. The personality and character of such stricken people needs nurture and the doctor, in his zeal to prolong life, must lessen as little as possible their zest for living. The personal physician from his place on a pedestal must replace some of the fears with hope—even when all seems hopeless—or he is no physician at all. In truth, my association with the incurably ill was an important part of my education as a human being.

As everyone knows, cancer is one of the major problems of medicine. Between 300 and 320 Canadians have cancer per

100,000 population. About 65,000 new cancer patients a year are diagnosed in our population of some 20 million—that is, about 3 new cases appear each year per 1,000 people. My associate and I in our last year of partnership (1953) identified 15 patients with cancer in a population of about 3,000. Judging by numbers, this is a small part of the work of a general practitioner, but the serious nature of the disease calls for an unending search for it as effective diagnostic procedures multiply and more types of cancer become amenable to improved treatment methods.

An incident early in my practice gave me much to think about. An elderly man returned after consulting at my direction a surgeon in London about a large mass in his abdomen. He brought with him a letter stating that he had an inoperable stomach cancer, and his general condition supported the verdict. He was very thin, unable to eat and in extreme misery with pain. He had now decided to see a herbalist in Kitchener, a quack with an enormous following.

I agreed. This was fine with me, I told him, but I wanted him to come in occasionally and tell me how he was getting along. He returned in two weeks, very pleased with himself. He had been assured that nothing was seriously the matter and was taking castor oil each morning with two ounces of whiskey before meals. He was now free of pain and eating everything, even beefsteak and onions. "Carry on, sir," was my advice. Two weeks later at 3 a.m. I was called to his home where he had died peacefully in his sleep.

Again I had to talk to myself. Here was a quack doing much more for an incurably ill man than I could. He had given him a month of comfortable living, when with me he couldn't eat. It wasn't the bit of alcohol the patient was taking that made him feel so much better. The hopeful attitude of his consultant was able somehow to strengthen the natural defense mechanisms of my patient's body and keep his cancer under better control. I didn't know that hope could bring such a transformation. To me this was a new dimension to treatment. It sounded very much like witchcraft or the ministrations of the shaman of primitive societies.

Another valuable lesson in understanding was afforded me by Tom who consulted me in my first year of practice. He was then a man in his fifties, so gaunt and pale that anyone could see at a glance he was ill. Examination disclosed a lump in his upper belly as large as my fist. What should I tell him in response to his plea that I be completely truthful? "I can take it," he assured me. So I gave him my verdict, that he probably had an incurable condition that warranted immediate further study. He thanked me, left and didn't return. Later I learned that a more understanding local physician took over his care. I say "more understanding" because I had been tricked into being too hasty. My conscience had made me inhumanely stupid. The realization was forced upon me that with the incurably ill I must be more perceptive in detecting how to encourage rather than alarm and so get their cooperation for further study and perhaps treatment.

In the case of John A. I employed more subtlety. He was a remarkable patient. He too came to me in an early year of practice, and he taught me so much that I must tell you a little about him. A businessman farmer with more than his share of success in both fields, he developed cancer of the rectum and both the consultant and I advised surgery. He stoutly refused. The prospect of a colostomy or bowel opening in his abdomen as a temporary measure horrified him. Moreover, this was such a new surgical procedure in 1924 that there were few patients anywhere who could testify to its value. It takes some years to popularize a new surgical procedure with other doctors and with patients.

John put me, his family physician, on a pedestal of hope—and woe betide me if I fell off by talking about his incurable ailment. To avoid this, we evolved a little game which went like this:

Occasionally on his visits to my office he would ask, "Friend Johnston (he never called me doctor), I am improving, am I not?"

"Yes, John," was always my answer.

Later, well along in his illness, I found that only morphine could give him much relief.

"Friend Johnston," he observed, "I hope there is nothing habit forming in these capsules."

"No. John, there is not." Of course, he knew differently.

"Then make them just a little stronger."

It was an April afternoon when John tottered into the office aided by his cane. He greeted me: "When the birds begin to sing and the grass gets green I'll be better, won't I?"

"Certainly, John."

A couple of hours later I had occasion to call on one of his close friends, the village clerk. "Doctor," he said, "your friend John is nearly done."

"Why do you say that?"

"He was in this afternoon after leaving your office and told me that 'when the grass gets green and the birds begin to sing, I will be under the sod'."

The final chapter was all his own. On an early June afternoon I was at his bedside when without any warning he remarked, "I understand you would like to go to Toronto next Monday for a three-day medical convention." Then he stuck out his skinny hand as he whispered, "I wish you to go. I won't be here when you come back, but I will be all right. Thanks for your wonderful help."

I could only thank him. He was gone when I returned.

As I said, John taught me much about the human race. He lived in the days when surgeons were perfecting their rather formidable operations for the removal of cancer of the rectum. In this atmosphere John refused to follow medical advice and proceeded to demonstrate how to end his days with dignity and without benefit of science, and how I as his personal doctor could aid him. He had no deep faith or traditional religion—he was just an ordinary person with a lot of courage.

On one occasion, after our dissembling remarks about his progress I became so concerned about the game we were playing that I approached his two sons. "Does your father appreciate the real nature of his affliction?" I asked them.

"Oh, certainly," they assured me. "His will is made and his business affairs are in order, with Mother provided for."

Dealing with his fears and depression was as important as my skill in meeting his physical disabilities. He packed into his body an indomitable will which enabled him to convert the horrors of an incurable illness into a challenge. I am reminded of a poem by the British poet William Ernest Henley:

Invictus

Out of the night that covers me,
Black as the pit from pole to pole,
I thank whatever gods may be
For my unconquerable soul.

In the fell clutch of circumstance
I have not winced nor cried aloud.
Under the bludgeonings of chance
My head is bloody, but unbow'd. . . .

It matters not how strait the gate,
How charged with punishments the scroll,
I am the master of my fate:
I am the captain of my soul.

These words were cerainly true of John, and were his personal banner.

Apropos this subject of bringing hope to the incurably ill, Dr. Dorothy Ley, a Toronto cancer specialist at Princess Margaret Hospital, made the following comment in 1968:

"Some doctors are keeping their cancer patients alive with large doses of personality; they are able to bolster the defence mechanism of the body in their patients to keep the disease under better control. Some patients whose disease has been kept under control by one doctor suffer serious relapses when treated by another doctor."

John looked life in the face and directed it right to the end.

He was one of many patients who did more for me than I could do for them. Human fearlessness of this nature often shows up unexpectedly. Reputedly strong men are frequently less able to face calmly their own demise than so-called weak individuals. Courage is like an iceberg—so much of it is hidden.

I am told there is a stained glass window at the Mayo Clinic in Rochester, Minnesota, with a panel showing Lister at work and bearing this motto: "To cure sometimes, to relieve often, to comfort always." It is something for every family doctor to keep in mind.

The various parts or tissues of our bodies are made up of building blocks called cells. Cancer cells are lawless; they grow like a disorderly mob. They invade normal surrounding body tissues in a unique and appalling manner. They never return to normal except when they occasionally disappear miraculously. We are in almost complete ignorance of how the normal body cell becomes cancerous and how it passes on its ungovernable powers of growth when dividing into two cells. Cancer kills one Canadian in six and deaths from it have not been significantly reduced in the last few decades.

So far as I can recollect, relatively few people with malignant disease consulted me in the 1920's, as compared with the numbers seen a couple of decades later. This paucity of cancer patients in the earlier days seems to be borne out by local statistics. The general hospital at Wingham, ten miles distant, had 183 medical and surgical admissions in 1920 and none was listed as a malignancy. I have no explanation for this.

And yet, in the 1920's there were always several people in the area with offensive looking lip cancers. Their occurrence was due largely to delay in consulting doctors because of scepticism about any kind of treatment. Some specialist surgeons of that date were very skillful in performing operations for lip cancer that involved widespread removal of neighboring glands. However, some of us felt these extensive procedures sometimes hastened the end of the patient instead of delaying it.

I referred early skin cancers to surgeons or excised them myself with a scalpel until about 1937 when diathermy machines with electro-coagulation needles became available along with the many other medical aids of that period. From then on I was able to cauterize these lesions so successfully that I ceased to refer them to others. There was the rare exception, as when the lesion occurred on an eyelid. I had only one recurrence, that of an early cancer of the upper lip. In this situation there were special hazards in treating with the electro-coagulation needle. The fee was five dollars. The same treatment was employed for early malignancies of the cervix, a part of the female genital tract readily reached with the electric needle. Internal cancers were a different matter.

It was impossible to predict how individuals would respond when confronted with the illness. Matthew, a farmer beyond middle age and with a grown family, was semi-retired. He was one of the salt of the earth and of the Methodist faith. I suspected a stomach malignancy and the x-ray proved it. He would go to Toronto only if I took him, so I did. On the way he asked; "How much will an operation cost, if the surgeon recommends it?"

"Ask him, he won't mind," I said.

We interviewed the late Dr. Roscoe Graham, a master craftsman of the art of medicine. He advised an operation, and in answer to Matthew's question he replied: "If you die during the the operation you will not be worried about money; if you live —and there is an 85 per cent chance of you doing so—please forget about money until you are well again, three or four months from now. At that time, come in and sit in that chair and we will discuss the fee. I promise you it will be acceptable to both of us."

Matthew and I returned home. On leaving him I urged that he make up his mind soon about having the operation.

"I will talk to the Lord and He will give me His answer," he promised.

"Please talk no longer than two weeks."

He took his time and came back in five weeks to announce, "I am now ready for the operation; it is the Lord's will."

Again I had to accompany him to the city. Dr. Graham—ever the gentleman—insisted that I scrub up and hold a retractor during the operation so that I could see what was going on. Matthew had a large stomach lesion at least two inches across. He returned home in about ten days.

"Matthew, did you have much pain?" I asked him.

This appeared to him a foolish question.

"None whatever. I knew before I went that I wouldn't have any."

I believed him and envied him his strong faith. He lived another ten years, the only patient with stomach cancer I ever knew to be apparently cured. I don't think this pleasing result had anything to do with his implicit trust in the Lord, but who knows for sure how far a completely serene mind can carry one?

A widow continued to live in the village after the death of her clergyman husband. She developed stomach symptoms, which became progressively worse. Before an exploratory operation was performed in a local hospital by a London surgeon she extracted a promise from me to tell her the full truth about our findings. It proved to be an inoperable growth. I was worried about my promise for I must never lie to patients and the immediate relatives must always know everything. The only relative this lady had in Canada was a sister in Montreal whom I did not know.

When I consulted my confrère, who had assisted at the operation, he replied, "Of course, you must keep your promise." Then the matron of the hospital, a quiet mature woman, came to my rescue by confiding, "Don't be so foolish. Your medical confrère didn't tell his own father last year under similar circumstances."

She was told that we found her trouble, that it might be serious and we would do the very best we could for her. She never enquired again. After her death I received a letter from her sister thanking me profusely for being so kind and including a cheque for fifty dollars over and above my fee—the only money gift I ever received.

My answer to this patient, with its triad of statements, became my stock answer to many hopeless patients: "We know your trouble and it may be serious, but we will do the best we can for you."

I never used the word cancer with these patients. Hope is a remarkable sustaining force and we ignore it at the risk of our patient's well-being. Everyone, and I mean everyone, wants to see the sun rise tomorrow. Some people, particularly the young, bravely insist that their doctor promise to tell them the whole truth and nothing but the truth when they become seriously ill. They know only partly whereof they speak They don't realize how much sick persons differ from well ones, just as sheep away from the flock are different sheep. Of course, my answer to the vexed question of how much to tell the hopelessly ill may not be the correct one for all doctors. Each physician must work out an answer of his own. I am telling you mine.

Donald was one of the village's most successful businessmen, who also travelled widely to address public meetings as an official promoter of the Dominion Government Annuities Pension Plan. He was past mid-life when he developed troublesome hip pain. The consultant I referred him to in Toronto bluntly informed him he had cancer of the prostate for which he could do little and prescribed x-ray therapy for the secondaries in his hip. Donald told me he put in a horrible six months adjusting to the idea that he must die soon. In a spirit of desperation, thinking to occupy his mind, he multiplied his speaking engagements, but even so he couldn't eat, sleep or properly concentrate and, in his words, he "went through hell."

To me the frankness of this consultant was most annoying. He was one whom I could never teach to stay away from dramatic pronouncements. Perhaps he was trying to show how competent and honest he was. Certainly he didn't appreciate that I, and not he, had to live with the patient. At the least, Donald's acute mental distress was unnecessary. He lived another five years and died suddenly of a stomach hemorrhage which may or may not have been associated with the malignancy. He should have been allowed to adjust himself slowly and without undue stress to early demise.

Harry too had cancer of the prostate. He came home to die after surgery and in the four months that followed my resources were taxed to their limit. Knowing how painful the illness was, I increased the frequency of my visits because I must not intensify his feeling of isolation and loneliness. A decrease of visits by a doctor through a distaste for the situation or a feeling of helplessness can be devastating to a patient. In this case we relieved the pain with aspirin, A.P.C.'s, morphine and its derivatives such as heroin, Nembutal and Pantopan. We induced sleep with alcohol, chloral, barbiturates and by trying to relieve anxiety and depression. Harry never discussed the nature of his illness and always ended my visit with the query, "How am I doing?" I learned to prepare for this question as soon as I entered his room. I would ask about everything I thought pertained to his welfare—eating, sleeping, the character of his pain, exercise, visitors, etc. Somewhere I would find some improvement since my last visit and this would constitute my reply. Of course, he recognized the game I was playing, but that was the way he wanted it.

I have stressed hope as the vital factor in the care of people with lengthy fatal illnesses. There are many other things that are important, such as a well-made bed, a well-managed bath, appetizing meals, the careful rationing of visitors, cheerful surroundings, the relief of pain, the privilege of sleeping as long as desired and the best place to spend the last days.

As for the best place for one to be in the case of terminal illness, most patients are happier in their homes provided they get adequate care. Mr. and Mrs. Thompson were in their forties and devoted to each other. He had an inoperable malignant disease and after a period in hospital wanted to remain at home. The problem was his increasing dependence on hypodermics for relief of pain and they could not afford twenty-four-hour nursing service. Mrs. Thompson shuddered at the thought of giving hypos, but was anxious to try.

"Why not get a plucked chicken and try giving it hypos of water?" I suggested, thinking this might faze her—it didn't. In a day she wanted to assume the responsibility of looking after her husband, and did so with amazingly successful results. Never have I known of an arrangement for a sick person's care at home to work out better.

Clarence had been in and out of hospital for leukemia and had reached the point where his life was being sustained almost solely by blood transfusions. In a frank discussion in hospital he gave me these instructions:

"As I am now dependent on blood transfusions at shorter and shorter intervals, I have discussed with my wife how we wish this to end. I would like now to go to our farm home and, if you agree, there will be no more transfusions."

I sent him home and both Clarence and his wife were grateful. As for me, I had no regrets. Clarence had every right to choose the manner of his dying, particularly when his choice was a carefully considered one.

Has a doctor the right to keep a man alive against his will and when he begs to be let go? Must the doctor always prolong the process of dying as long as possible? Or, to put it another way, should he allow a person in his care to die several times? I am just asking.

The experiences recounted in this chapter occurred in the period 1920 to 1940. Later on, in the 1950's, it became more difficult to decide when to stop active treatment of the hopelessly ill people. Such measures as intravenous feedings and better sedation made it much easier to prolong the lives of the incurably ill without severe discomfort to them. More children wanted to keep father and mother living until the last moment. Hospital nursing staffs seemed more zealous about getting the reputation of doing everything possible for the sick. Doctors in general seemed more reluctant to "step back and let God take over," as Dr. Walter C. Alvarez, a former Mayo Clinic specialist, has put it.

In this discussion I have dwelt rather long on the therapy effects of the physician himself as friend, adviser and comforter. The problem of what to tell the patient with cancer today has markedly changed from that of the 1930's and 1940's because modern medical care with its special hospitals, radio therapy, improved surgery, hormones and chemotherapy can do much more for him than was ever possible before. However, the rôle of the physician himself as a therapeutic agent will continue to be a paramount one.

It is proper to insist that the earlier people report suspicious symptoms to their doctor the greater is their chance for successful treatment, should the trouble prove to be malignant. But it is wrong to give assurance that early diagnosis is a guarantee of cure. Despite this caution, there have been so many positive and realistic advances in the field of cancer that our citizens have every inducement to trust today's physicians and to be as liberal as possible with donations to help research. Certainly more and more research is urgently needed to meet some of the grim statistics. For instance, we were told in 1971: a) that a patient with symptomatic lung cancer has only a 10 per cent chance of surviving five years after treatment has started; b) that the five-year survival rate of osteogenic sarcoma (bone cancer) is a dismal 17 per cent even with amputation.

True, there are no guarantees. Yet there is much to make one optimistic that a breakthrough toward mastery of this dread disease may not be far away if we keep searching.

XI. Old Scourges Have Gone—Some Remain

It is curious, looking back, to recall the diseases that once produced terror and today are seldom heard of.

There was diphtheria. Not many decades ago it was a bane of Canadian communities. My father, about 1880, saw two of his sisters die from it in the same week. They were the strongest members of the family. Yet in my years of practice I encountered only three children with it. They were in their early teens and members of the same family. They did not appear very ill, though each had a temperature of 101°, a racing pulse and a peculiar distinctive odor to the breath. With the help of diphtheria antiserum they were well in a few days. I always carried throat swab tubes in my bag and had a supply of diphtheria antitoxin and antiserum in my office refrigerator. The breakthrough for this disease had come in 1913 when Bela Schick, the Hungarian-born allergist, devised the skin test which bears his name.

I saw in my time only one patient with scurvy, a plump seven-month-old child of a prosperous farm family. The baby was ill in the winter months with bleeding gums and the large thigh blood clot of a full-blown scurvy. It was a bottle-fed baby.

Scurvy is due to a vitamin C deficiency. Dependable dietary sources of this vitamin are the citrus fruits, green leaf vegetables, Irish potatoes, and tomatoes, some of which were scarce in winter months before the days of modern transportation and storage. The French-Canadian pioneers in our country feared this late winter scourge and sometimes drank a brew made by boiling young evergreen branches. During the era of sailing ships the British Admiralty added lemons to the diet of sailors as soon as it was discovered empirically that lemon juice prevented the ailment. It was from the lemons in the diet of the British sailor that he got his nickname "limey," bestowed by Americans. Limehouse takes its name from the wharf where the lemons were stored. Curiously, Sicilian and Mediterranean lemons are effective, but for some unknown reason West Indian lemons are nearly inert.

Rickets, a disease due primarily to the lack of Vitamin D, was once common among children, but that was before my day. It may be mild or severe, its symptoms varying from mere irritability in the child and a few physical signs to widespread bone deformities. Although I didn't identify a single case of any type, it is occasionally seen today in the Sick Children's Hospital in Toronto. It may be present as a tetany and premature infants are especially prone to it. Most milk sold commercially is, of course, fortified with vitamin D. Exposure to sunlight and vitamin D, along with a balanced diet, are curative.

Nor did I encounter a single patient with typhoid fever. We saw a number with para-typhoid, a much milder disease. One was a middle-aged man whom we operated on for appendicitis. He presented difficulties in diagnosis both to me and the surgeon because this illness was so rare. It took this unfortunate man six to eight weeks to recover completely from his para-typhoid fever plus the surgery.

Instead of typhoid fever we had undulant fever to puzzle us with its swinging temperature that persisted for weeks. It was quite a common ailment in the thirties. As is well known today, it comes from drinking raw milk from cows infected with contagious abortion, or brucellosis. Before reliable diagnostic tests were discovered patients frequently went for weeks undiagnosed. It was finally controlled by eliminating the disease in cattle and by the introduction of pasteurized milk. Also some helpful antibiotics appeared on the market.

Infectious mononucleosis was another puzzling ailment. It was first named in 1920 and appeared to practicing doctors as a completely new disease—one we had not heard about before.

The diarrheal diseases, so prevalent in the twenties (see Chapter VII) have given way to accidents as the most common cause of children's deaths today. Nevertheless, although these diseases are no longer as familiar as they once were, Dr. Harry Bain of the Sick Children's Hospital at Toronto, reports that they are still a serious child's ailment there. The treatment, as in the 1940's, is as much fluid as possible in as many ways as possible. Occasionally from culturing bowel movements they find salmonella organisms, but it is believed now that 90 per cent of children's serious diarrhea disorders are due to viruses. As a result antibiotics are of little aid in combating them. They await better treatment measures.

Scabies or itch, a skin disease due to an animal parasite which buries under the epidermis, was a common troublesome complaint we have almost forgotten—not death-dealing, but its intolerable itching could play havoc with whole families. Our treatment was the application of 10 per cent precipitated sulphur ointment until the introduction of Benzyl Benzoate in 1937, which proved so effective we thought we had the ailment completely mastered. Certainly we saw fewer patients with it. But in 1970 some Ontario doctors reported a remarkable increase in the incidence of scabies infestation, along with the fact that the disease seemed more resistant to the old standard treatment. So perhaps we are not yet through with it.

In my early years many parents thought their children weren't properly prepared for adult life unless they had suffered from whooping cough, measles, mumps and chicken pox. Some mothers even deliberately exposed their children to these ailments in the belief that they were milder illnesses in childhood than in grown-ups.

Whooping cough was a common ailment. Hospital authorities used to report a 50% mortality rate under one year of age. I recollect only one death and that in a child of three years soon after pneumonia developed as a complication. Now there is a vaccine with an efficacy rate of 80 to 85 per cent and there are now few deaths.

There is now a good vaccine against measles which confers a lasting immunity. I saw no fatalities from this disease.

Mumps was and remains a common ailment. There was no preventative for mumps until a vaccine was introduced early in 1972 by the Connaught Laboratories.

In today's terminology, these are largely "old-fashioned" diseases that have been responsive to the new medical advances. Research workers of this century have discovered an amazing variety of measures for healthier living, ranging all the way from vaccines and vitamins to hundreds of antibiotics for checking hundreds of kinds of infections. But the task is far from completed. Major ailments remain for mankind to master that have yielded little or not at all to modern drugs and techniques.

One of these is heart disease. It is sad indeed to see so many men and women in their forties and early fifties laid low today with heart attacks, people in the very prime of life. Many dedicated physicians and surgeons are imaginative and fearless in developing new techniques to repair the damaged coronary arteries and to supply heart transplants, yet the realization that we know very little about the prevention of these disasters confronts us as a constant challenge.

A second major killer of mankind, of course, is cancer. Most external cancers are under control, but many internal ones baffle us. Among the many exciting developments in the cancer field, not the least is the launching of a great national effort by President Richard Milhouse Nixon and the American Congress to find "a cure" for the disease. And the teams of research workers closing in on the secrets of cancer growth and therapy for its control also give us reason to hope. One such research project, under the direction of Dr. Isaac Djerassi of the United States, is reported by Stewart Alsop in an interesting interview in the December 1971 issue of *Newsweek*.

Our bone marrow is our blood factory and a person is said to have leukemia when his bone marrow is attacked by cancer cells. To treat the condition powerful chemicals are introduced into his veins to prolong his life. There are three kinds of good blood cells—red cells which give us life by carrying oxygen and other substances, platelets which prevent us from bleeding to death, and white cells which fight infection. Blood transfusions, introduced about 1900, were the first true body transplants. Because many leukemia patients being treated by helpful chemicals die from hemorrhages, Dr. Djerassi helped to develop the technique of giving them transfusions of concentrated solutions of blood platelets. But although this decreased the tendency to hemorrhage, many of the leukemia patients have responded by dying of infections. Dr. Djerassi is now perfecting a method of giving billions of white cells in concentrated solution as a transfusion. This is expected to be a boon to patients suffering from leukemia as well as to others, including those with lung and bone cancers.

Researchers now seem convinced that there will be no simple single cure developed for all cancers, but rather two hundred or so different cures for as many kinds of cancer. It seems probable that today's surgery and x-ray therapy for cancer may soon be replaced by chemotherapy and immunotherapy. This optimism is warranted by the large number of individual intuitive cancer researchers like Dr. Djerassi at work on the problem.

Still another serious ailment awaiting a breakthrough in our knowledge is the family of ills that include arthritis, rheumathoid arthritis and the plain old complaint known as rheumatism. These are not so much killers as misery-producers to countless people. From personal experience I am acquainted with arthritis. Of course, we can do a lot to relieve the arthritic.

At one time, it was hoped that a cure for arthritis had been found with the discovery of cortisone in 1948. A new page in medical history was written when Dr. Philip Hench of the Mayo Clinic gave a new drug, Compound E (cortisone) to a bedridden, crippled, pain-wracked woman with arthritis. The patient's swollen joints subsided miraculously and in three days she was out of bed and shopping downtown.

Resting on the top of each of our kidneys is a small gland called the adrenal gland weighing a quarter of an ounce. The central part of each gland, its medulla, secretes a hormone called "adrenalin," and known since 1895. The cortex or outer rind of each gland produces other hormones called steroids or corticosteroids. Some persistent scientists, among whom were Doctors Edward Kendall and Lewis Sarett of the Mayo Clinic, starting with several tons of animal adrenal glands, extracted steroids from their cortex which they named alphabetically beginning with Compound A.

Compound A was worthless, Compond E was named cortisone. Compound F became the first improved cortisone and was called hydro-cortisone. It was followed by an even better one called Prednisone. The first cortisone produced cost $200 a gram and was worth 175 times its weight in gold. It was early prepared from ox bile and later from the roots of a Mexican vine.

But early hopes that cortisone was a cure for arthritis were soon dashed. The drug relieved the symptoms of arthritis miraculously, but it didn't cure. Disturbing side effects sometimes appeared and occasionally it seemed to cause flare-ups of tuberculosis, diabetes and stomach ulcers. Nevertheless, more than 150 wide-ranging illnesses have proven to be amenable to treatment with synthetic steroids. One of these is acute cortical adrenal insufficiency characterized by a sudden dramatic collapse, as shown in the following two cases recorded by Dr. Murray Fisher, a general practitioner in Gravenhurst, Ontario.

"In 1945 I saw a 44-year old female patient with moderately severe low abdominal pain. It was fairly easy to reach a diagnosis of ovarian cyst with a twisted pedicle. A competent surgeon removed it in hospital. The operation was without any untoward incident and the patient was in good post-operative condition.

"All went well until the fourth day when at an early morning visit in response to an emergency call, I found an unbelievable change in the patient. She was utterly prostrated with a feeble pulse and a blood pressure so low it was almost impossible to determine. In consultation with the surgeon we were satisfied there was no internal bleeding, but we were at a complete loss to explain the picture. She died in a few hours. Permission for an autopsy was refused.

"Five years later, in 1950 another female patient was brought into the office at 5 p.m. Her husband helped to carry her in. I quickly recognized the picture I had seen previously; she was in the same state of extreme collapse, the same feeble pulse. In this case there was something added. She was bronzed all over. It was summer and I almost mistook her facial color for a suntan.

"I gave her a vial of Solu Cortef (Upjohn) intravenously. In the local hospital I got intravenous fluids started. She responded well, and I gave her more Solu Cortef to maintain her blood pressure. In the morning she was on her way to the Toronto General Hospital where a diagnosis of acute adrenal insufficiency was confirmed. This is sometimes called Addison's Disease. She was put on cortisone by mouth and returned home in a month in fair condition and remained on it as long as I had any contact with her."

The first patient in 1945 died as there was no cortisone while the second in 1950 recovered due to the fortunate discovery of the drug in 1948.

Aspirin remains the main pain reliever for arthritis with the newer enteric-coated ones supposedly free from any stomach irritants; also Butazolidin and indocid have some curative powers. Many hospitals now have physiotherapy departments with local heat facilities for these patients and with exercise programs, which are painful—but pain is the name of the game. A few lucky arthritics can spend a period in the warm dry climate of Tucson, Arizona. Furthermore, merchants are coming forward with many helpful aids, such as electric blankets, long-handled shoe horns and elastic shoe laces. Yet with all this we are woefully lacking in basic knowledge of the fundamental causes of arthritis and the best means of preventing it.

Then there is the problem of the addictions, still the strangest of all maladies. An addiction may be defined as an overpowering impulse to take into the body a substance possessing soothing or intoxicating properties. Nicotine and alcohol are as surely addictive as drugs, and physicians' attitudes to their overuse reflects in part society's perplexing experiences with addicts and government's uncertain attempts to impose regulations.

Take the problem of addiction to nicotine through prolonged cigarette smoking. Why are so many people loath to pay attention to the careful studies of the rôle of cigarette smoking in causing lung cancer? I shudder a little every time I see a young, robust and healthy-looking person take out his package of Cameo's or Sweet Caporals preparatory to lighting up. It is such a hazardous pleasure. The statistic is: start smoking at 20 and smoke 20 or more cigarettes a day and your insurance company will lose because on the average your life expectation is reduced eight years; someone with a yen for figures estimates that this means your life is shortened 14.4 minutes per cigarette. Of course, this is just an average—you may live longer or you may die some years short of the average.

Over the last thirty-five years deaths from lung cancer have shown a fifteen-fold increase in men. Emphysema became five times more common in the 1953-1963 decade. In 1971 the estimated new cases in Canada were male 3800, female 700—and they were largely preventable. The figures are alarming, in this country and elsewhere, and it is further cause for dismay that much of the increase in deaths from lung cancer is said by authorities in this field to be due to cigarette smoking.

As I said in an earlier chapter, all the narcotic addicts I saw in the 1920's were morphine addicts. Today studies show that 90 per cent of narcotic addicts are heroin users. We are with good reason alarmed by this, and by the increasing popularity of the newer addictive agents such as the amphetamines, LSD and glue, and possibly marijuana. Yet the most common addiction is still the overuse of alcohol.

It seems to me—I may be wrong in this—that some segments of the medical profession are pessimistic about ever finding a cure for alcoholism. Now that it is recognized as an illness, perhaps what we need is not a cure so much as we need prevention. Mankind has mastered few, if any, of its afflictions by treatment, yet it has learned how to control scores of them by prevention.

Alcoholism involves three factors: the substance itself, the individual, and society. It is in the interaction of these three elements that the problem occurs, so it must be in the balancing of them that the primary prevention of alcoholism can be effected. Because it is such a complex illness and an involved public health problem we need a wide-open frame of mind when considering the long-term goal. By "primary prevention" I mean taking steps which will inform non-drinkers and help new drinkers especially to become aware of the effects of alcohol in various quantities so that they will be able to gauge their capacity and avoid the dangers of drinking too much too often. The aim of secondary prevention is to reduce the number of alcoholics by finding them early and treating them.

Treatment holds no final answers. The only hope of getting at the root problem of chronic undisciplined drinking lies in education and legislation. It is the business of all concerned citizens, calling for the cooperation of parents, teachers, clergy, medical people and other adults in charting ways to live more safely in our alcohol-oriented society.

The extent of the problem is suggested by a study reported in 1968, by the Addiction Research Foundation of Ontario. Their elaborate findings on the consumption of beverage alcohol in Ontario revealed that in a population of five million people fifteen years of age and older, probably 72 per cent were drinkers. The amount of whiskey or its equivalent consumed daily per person varied, it was estimated, between one ounce or less and forty ounces. More specifically, graphs following a normal logarithmic curve showed that 400,000 adults consumed 2-3 ounces of whiskey a day; more than 100,000 consumed 10-15 ounces; 22,750 consumed 20-25 ounces. And so on.

It is not difficult to appreciate the difference between the many who drank 5 ounces or less of liquor daily and the smaller group of approximately 60,000 who drank in excess of 20 ounces. The latter were either grossly intoxicated at frequent intervals or in a continuous state of mild intoxication.

When does consumption become dangerous? Some scientists have placed the danger point at five gallons absolute alcohol yearly or about six ounces of whiskey daily. Others have placed it at nine gallons yearly or about ten ounces daily.

Whatever the case, the present distribution of consumption shows that a substantial number of Ontario drinkers consume alcoholic beverages in quantities hazardous to health. And there is no reason to believe that the habits of Ontario citizens are peculiar in this regard, judged by social standards throughout the Western world.

To tackle the problem of dependence upon alcohol we need answers to some basic questions. Why do people in good health drink, and what leads them to drink to excess? We need to know more about this. Because they like it, is not answer enough. All of them do not drink just to get a warm glow. And it is far too trite and fusty an answer to say that all alcoholics began excessive drinking as an escape or refuge from life's miseries and worries. Everyone has anxieties. "Anxiety" and "stress" are two of the most overworked words of our time. They occur whenever an individual is in conflict with himself, and such conflicts are not all harmful. No one has shown that men are more subject to anxiety than women, yet there are six times as many male alcoholics as female in our society.

The Bible tells us that Noah planted a vineyard and became drunk—thereby establishing the respectable antiquity of fermented liquor. In more recent days there were the Saxons with their flowing cups of mead, and our own pioneers who relied on alcohol to lighten the miseries and discomforts of opening up the wilderness. Its mystical properties have been lauded (often) by people of genuine creative gifts who claim that it stimulates the intellect, enlarges the consciousness, serves to erase timidity and act as a tranquillizer. Some have found it satisfying because it allows them temporarily to disown their burdens and achieve an illusory security. Jack London, Brendan Behan, Dylan Thomas, Damon Runyon and Sir Winston Churchill were among those who found liquor supportive, an aid to creativity. Surely such long-term usage is argument that it must meet some basic need and not be a wholly unmitigated evil. The fact that at least 90 per cent of those who drink beverage alcohol do not suffer from alcoholism reinforces the view that it helps many more people than it damages.

The persons damaged, and their numbers are large enough, create the problem. To approach it we must reach a fuller understanding of what is good and what is bad about alcohol usage—and what is hoary myth. The new concept of alcoholism as an illness has been enormously effective in providing a more tolerant and humane atmosphere for discussion. And one result is that we now look for alcoholics in new places. The problem is no longer confined to the low-paid so-called lower classes drinking gin and falling down in the gutter, but extends to the highly paid business executives who are never quite sober, never quite drunk, just high on expensive cocktails and spirits. There are the social pressures to drink excessively and a tolerance of drunken behavior to be taken into account.

Other basic questions beg for answers. For instance: What is safe drinking, or is none of it safe? Is it our object to make our children live without alcohol, or to use it in moderation if they choose to drink?

A major part of the responsibility to provide education in the use of alcohol rests upon parents, many of whom may fear to tread here. They may be embarrassed, too emotionally involved, or may simply not have the knowledge to impart. They may know how to drink themselves but have not given thought to instructing their children. Parents are not in a strong position to moralize—only to inform. We can trust young people if we provide them with knowledge. Those of today have more information than any generation before them. I sympathize with the young man who observed that he wouldn't be proud to say at the end of his day, "I have never taken a drink." On the other hand, I have only respect for the sincere prohibitionists; studies show that where abstinence is the prevailing attitude of a group, alcoholism is relatively rare among its members.

Orthodox Jews associate much of their drinking with meals and religious observances in which the children participate and yet with these people drunkenness is frowned upon and alcoholism is rare. There is a lesson here for many parents.

We start with the premise that every adult has two rational

choices—total abstinence or moderate controlled drinking, meaning drinking that is appropriate to the time, the place and the person. Youth is searching for attitudes, values and meaningful relationships in every department of life. These are ageless quests. The basic issue is sensible and responsible behavior, not simply the avoidance of what may be harmful—to learn how to get the most out of life, how to enrich and strengthen ourselves and others, how to make morally right and socially responsible decisions. Whether or not we use alcoholic beverages is a very secondary consideration. Drinking cannot be isolated as an activity in itself. What could be done by a teenager in the 1930's as a rebel and deviant might be done by a teenager in the 1960's and '70's as a conformist. Such are the current changes in attitude. Self-responsibility and self-identity in the use of alcohol are a part of the realities of living.

The physician is in a unique position to help with the drinking problem on an individual basis but he cannot expect to accomplish much if he neglects to give thought to the society of which the individual is a part—to his family, community, job relationships. It may be said of alcoholism what Sir William Osler said of tuberculosis, that it is "a social disorder with medical aspects."

Youth is the time to instil needed controls, and the concerted efforts of influential people in all walks of community life—including members of Alcoholics Anonymous—can bring about a reduction in alcohol dependence and addiction. This is not easily accomplished today by prohibition, but rather by personal example, understanding and sympathetic firmness. Enterprising admen try to convince the public that with every bottle of liquor we purchase we are buying companionship, relaxation, vigor, special moments, goodwill and glitter. These are half-truths, but it is too much to expect the advertisers to volunteer words of caution. It is up to the rest of us to sell to the young the idea that the stimulation and goodwill flowing from alcohol are best accompanied by sobriety and reason.

I will venture stating two conclusions which seem to me inescapable. First, to decrease the number of alcoholics entering our society each year, we must somehow reduce our total consumption of alcoholic beverage. Second, this means we must meet the problem of cutting down the prevalence of social drinking. Every alcoholic was once a moderate social drinker. This will be really a touchy and ticklish task calling for much careful thinking by both our young people and our adults.

In a review of what has been accomplished by medical science in my time and what remains to challenge the profession in future, it is necessary to comment more fully on the remarkable advances made in understanding and treating the mentally retarded. For me, it has been one of the happiest developments of recent decades—though, admittedly, there is still much to be learned and much to be done in promoting new attitudes toward this old and potentially tragic human condition.

Of all the cares and anxieties of life, few can compare with those of a mother having charge of a retarded child. Yet, in the 1920's, the mentally retarded and feebleminded were ignored by both the medical profession and the public. There was little interest in them anywhere. Dr. Alan Brown, Chief of the Hospital for Sick Children in Toronto, paid little attention to them, in his book *Common Procedures in the Practice of Paediatrics*, which was written in 1932. Of the mongoloid he says only that they usually die during the first two years of life from bronchopneumonia and that no treatment improves the condition. The experts of that day held that intelligence was fixed at birth, that the causes of brain defects were genetic and that our chief hope was to prevent the birth of more defective people.

I recall a feeble-minded girl living into her mid-twenties, confined in a child's playpen in a farmhouse kitchen. She couldn't feed or dress herself. She was always babbling away and playing with a simple toy. She was untidy and unkempt, but close observation showed that her parents and one brother gave immediate and unceasing attention to her every wish and whim. The parents steadily refused to send her to a mental hospital, the only residential care institution then available for such a person.

Another retarded girl was a member of a clergyman's family

of four children. After much discussion and soul-searching the parents had her admitted to the Ontario mental hospital in Orillia, which was for the insane and seriously disturbed.

In the twenties the idea of teaching the feeble-minded was ridiculed as a useless labor and extravagance. Because a defective learns slowly, many were misled into believing they could not learn at all. Then with the establishment in 1958 of the Ontario Association for the Care of the Feeble-minded the atmosphere surrounding these people changed profoundly, with one progressive move following another in quick succession.

The old classification of the feeble-minded into morons, imbeciles and idiots gradually became outdated. The subnormal child is now considered by authorities to differ only in degree and not in kind from the normal and superior; the points of resemblance are much greater than the differences. Teachers now emphasize these similarities and try to make the environment of the subnormal child as close as possible to that of the normal child.

A recent brochure published by the Canadian Association for the Care of the Mentally Retarded is helpful in defining the condition and correcting widespread misconceptions about it.

By mental retardation is meant impaired mental ability. The mentally retarded have the minds of children, regardless of age; at maturity the capacity to understand will be less than normal. Mental defect and mental illness are not to be confused. They are entirely distinct and one does not lead to the other. Mental illness consists in disordered functioning of the mind, while retardation indicates a lack of intelligence. It has come to be measured in terms of intelligence-quotient, commonly referred to as I.Q. In these terms the mildly retarded child is generally defined within the I.Q. range of 50-70; the moderately retarded 35-50; the severely retarded 20-35 and the profoundly retarded below 20. An intelligence-quotient of 90-100 is the range of ordinary or "average" minds. It is fair to say that some authorities view this I.Q. classification of the mentally retarded as rather irrelevant.

Of the two hundred known causes of retardation (in many

cases the cause is still unknown) the commonest are: an imperfect or damaged brain, because of something wrong with the chromosomes of the parents, or something affecting the mother's health during pregnancy, or damage while the child is being born; and bad living conditions with neglect or mistreatment of the baby, which can interfere with the development of its brain. There is still much to be done in discovering and dealing with the causes of retardation.

No family is immune. An accident of nature, birth injury or a disease in infancy can strike any home and any family of every class and race—rich and poor, learned and ignorant. It is not curable because it is not a disease but a life-long condition. There are some conditions, however, resembling mental retardation which can be improved or cured. For instance, deafness, poor vision, emotional disturbance or poor living conditions may sometimes make a normal child appear retarded. All children, therefore, who seem backward should be carefully investigated, to discover if possible the reason for their slow development.

I recall a child of six years in a family of seven children who was considered mentally retarded until specialist examination revealed that she had defective vision. On treatment of this impairment there was a dramatic improvement in her learning capacity. In fact, she spoke her first words the day after she was given glasses.

It may come as a surprise that mental retardation is the commonest of all childhood disabilities. Three out of every hundred children born are mentally retarded to some degree. Contrary to the general belief that the condition is hopeless, twenty-nine out of thirty of them can be helped to grow into useful happy members of the community, with a considerable degree of self-sufficiency. But the retarded child and his family need early expert counselling in getting used to the handicap.

The mildly retarded—those who have not suffered more than about twenty-five per cent mental impairment below normal intelligence—can with proper teaching succeed in school work from the second to sixth grade range. These are the "educable" retarded, who represent nearly 83 per cent of all mentally retarded. Twenty-five out of thirty retarded children are educable and can be taught to be fairly self-supporting as adults. Another 13 per cent, or four out of every thirty, are moderately retarded and are classed as "trainable." With proper schools and sheltered workshops they can become self-supporting to some degree. One child in thirty is severely retarded and may need life-long nursing care. Such children are the "dependent." Research is now finding methods of helping even the severely handicapped to achieve hitherto unexpected levels of self-help.

Indicative of what is being done for those children, there are now twenty large public residential establishments for the mentally retarded across Canada, totalling about sixteen thousand beds and served by a staff of over six thousand. Ontario has four of these so-called hospital schools, which authorities consider schools rather than hospitals, at Smiths Falls, Orillia, Cedar Springs in the London area, and Palmerston. In addition, the province now has many smaller community residences for the mentally retarded which are gaining in popularity.

In a brochure entitled "The Mentally Handicapped Child," Dr. H. F. Frank, a past medical superintendent of the Smiths Falls Hospital School, offers this caution to parents of mentally handicapped children living at home:

"It is not enough to know that a child is mentally handicapped. He may be mentally like an average infant; or like an average child approaching maturity. A mildly handicapped child will be like average children from 8 to 12 years. A moderately handicapped one will be like average children from 3 to 7 years and the severely handicapped are those who, when adult, will have the mental capacity of the average child not over three years. A point often overlooked yet important is that while some one or two per cent of the population are mentally handicapped, a much larger number have only borderline intelligence. Members of this group are frequently troublesome as borderline types do not fit well at school or at work, with the normal or the mentally handicapped."

In general, it is agreed that the majority of mentally retarded children get along well in a community and only a small percentage require institutional care. Especially in the case of the very young, institutional care may not be wise unless a multiple handicap is present. The idea that most mental defectives are delinquent, even degenerate, has proven to be false. They are seldom the instigators of serious crimes but are usually led into trouble by their brighter companions.

In this field, as in so many others, the challenge to further investigation is great, the need urgent. But doors have opened and exciting progress is being made.

A few words on the subject of geriatrics, an area in which many family doctors find their greatest social rôle.

Someone has said, "after 60 years you are going down hill no matter how well you feel." The most common afflictions of the elderly are loneliness, forgetfulness and deafness. A considerable number of the elderly are stricken with the triad of symptoms of dizziness, deafness and ringing in the ears known as the Menières Syndrome. This can be so alarming to the victim that he is sure he is having a stroke. "Strokes," heart attacks, and mental depressions are also all too frequent.

Most old people urgently need the attention of friends and the more the better, and yet how prone many young folk are to mistakenly send Father and Mother to locations where they have no acquaintances whatever. We urgently need research to find out who should be in nursing homes, what their health needs are, and how these needs can be met.

In treating the chronically ill and elderly patients, we need competent leadership based on wide experience and much sympathy. Fortunately this year Ontario is establishing a network of nursing homes right across the province. This revolutionary program should help assure a more valuable and perhaps even more pleasant old age for our citizens.

As Cicero put it, "allow us to learn in good time the principle by which we may easily support the weight of increasing years."

XII. A Glance into the Future of Family Medicine

Let us look briefly at the future of the general practitioner-family doctor, with special reference to the Canadian experience. I give him this hyphenated title because it more completely describes him in his rôle as a community family doctor. I shall not try to look very far into the future, just around the nearest corner, as I have no ability in reading palms or teacups, and little gift of forecasting. I found even the simple exercise of foretelling the demise of a hopelessly ill patient so chancy that I early ceased to attempt it. Moreover, many men much wiser than I have made themselves ridiculous by their false prognostications.

In 1860 the French chemist, Marcel Berthelot, said: "Within a hundred years of physical and chemical science man will know what the atom is. It is my belief that when science reaches this age God will come down to earth with his big ring of keys and will say to humanity 'Gentlemen, it is closing time.'" The late Walter Reuther is reported to have said, "Science could bring paradise to earth by the year 2000," to which Dr. Billy Graham replied, "There is a flaw here. No one has fed into the computers the facts about man's moral weakness, his tendency toward hate, lust and greed that produce racism, crime, war and a thousand other evils." Such remarks reflect a little mankind's insatiable desire to know the future and suggest what widely different views thoughtful people can hold.

So much has been written recently about the care doctors and their helpers are giving the sick and injured, about the controversial issue of the vanishing general practitioner and the urgent need for more personal treatment, that I ask: Is there anything more to say? I think there is—not because of me, who at seventy-four cannot be vain, but because of the inexhaustible nature of the subject and people's unquenchable interest in their health.

Whither Caduceus? This exercise of peering even cautiously ahead presents baffling problems. There is such steady and astounding progress in medical science as well as in society that we have scarcely time to assess one change before another is upon us. People are living longer so there is the paradoxical phenomenon of more elderly folk in our communities along with an increasing percentage of young people. We are all living less and less isolated lives now that we can be anywhere in the world in a few hours. And, finally, government has become a firm partner in medicine, with new instalments of pre-paid government health-insurance plans appearing every month or so.

As for the general practitioner, his image—and how I mistrust that word—declined steadily through the 1930's to 1950's, until the point was reached where the respected and beloved family doctor of old was becoming in the eyes of the public a professional incompetent concerned first with personal gain and only secondarily with the welfare of the sick. Moreover, so few young doctors were choosing general practice as a career that the family doctors still practicing in town and city were dangerously overworked; many communities found themselves without any physician at all. The situation was so serious that both the medical profession and the laity were asking in innumerable articles the questions: Is there a place for the general practitioner in the future health-care structure? If there is, what will his position be?

The complaints about the care being given by general-practitioner—family doctors were many:

First of all, they erected barriers to protect themselves:

a) by installing telephone answering services which are unyielding in shielding the doctor from patient intrusion;

b) by making a practice of having unlisted home telephone numbers;

c) eliminating house calls, even for emergencies, which effectively cuts the doctor off from whole categories of ill people;
d) making themselves unavailable after office hours, over weekends and on the mid-week golf day; and
e) employing helpers who shield the doctor from pestering patients.

Such measures were adopted in the name of more efficient and improved practice. Of course they were defensive in order to lessen the pressures of crushing overwork and to insure that the doctors could perform reasonable services and still have time for rest and relaxation with their families.

The truth is that gradually Canada became seriously short of an adequate number of doctors. Dr. Harry Roberts, 1971-72 President of the Canadian Medical Association, reports our medical schools are putting out only 1000 students a year when we need 2000; in 1970 Ontario trained 340 doctors and imported 582, and British Columbia graduated 52, a ratio of one graduate per 41,000 population, whereas the Canadian average is one graduate per 20,000.

Secondly, doctors were further accused of maintaining a medical organization which to many people appeared to be of the antiquated guild-type wherein the needs of patients were subordinated to their own well-being, and within its sheltering confines the profession seemed to close ranks to protect its members in trouble.

The concept of community control of community health is a development of the time and disturbs a substantial part of the medical profession which is convinced that physicians should control the structure of health services because of their greater knowledge in this field. But the public is the final arbiter and will eventually get the health care it wants because it pays the bills.

Thirdly, doctors were accused of over-emphasizing the acquisition of money; of worshipping the call of the Golden Fleece; of making medicine more and more a business and less and less a profession.

From my observations I would agree that the chief ambition of many young doctors today seems to be to own a house, car and summer cottage, all paid for within the first five years of practice—whereas we oldsters looked upon this as a lifetime task. I may be unfair in this assessment of my younger confrères. Nonetheless, despite my advancing years, I judge my sensory organs to remain reasonably perceptive and as such detect an increased concern for more almighty dollars, a concern prompted by what some euphemistically call enlightened self-interest.

Finally the public questioned the assertion of physicians that in medical matters they are competent judges of their own capabilities and limitations. It disturbed many people that they were too much at the mercy of the doctors and must accept their concept of themselves—which was to say that there was too little professional supervision of doctors' work. The truth, of course, is that few people are blessed with sound insight into their own abilities.

There was some justice in many of these charges, but by far the most serious situation was that medical schools were not equipping students with the broad knowledge and experience to qualify them as competent family doctors. Here are a few of the common ailments neglected by medical school curricula:

1. There was no attention to psychiatry as we understand it today. The only psychiatry taught in medical schools of the 1920's and 30's pertained to those with serious mental illnesses and the insane. This may be called major psychiatry. There was nothing for the worried and anxious, the emotionally disturbed, what we might call minor psychiatry. Young doctors on graduation were amazed to find that the worried and anxious constituted about twenty-five percent of their patients and they were ill-prepared to meet them. They found whole families of nervous and frightened people. They had to learn unaided how to make contact with the personalities lurking behind the common complaints of headache, backache, and dyspepsia.

2. A grave oversight was the lack of training in massage and

manipulation for injured muscles, tendons, and joints without fractures present. For instance, a sprain of the sacro-iliac joint of the lower back is a common disability. I tried different types of manipulation for this—a few helped, but most didn't, and when desperate I referred them to a district osteopath whom I had learned to trust. I envied him what he could do for such sprains and felt let down in this by my teachers. I should have been able to do as much as, and even more than, osteopaths: we general practitioners had more going for us.

Osteopaths are well-trained doctors. They operate over three hundred osteopathic hospitals in the United States, many of them maintaining intern and residency training programs. Osteopathic medicine has copied much of the structure of orthodox medicine and one of its aims is to make the patient feel more secure.

Osteophathic massage and manipulation undoubtedly do improve the overall health of people. Osteopaths maintain this is true in the presence of many diseases such as diabetes, stomach ulcers, sinus infections and even pneumonia. In adopting massage and manipulation as treatment modalities, conventional medicine does not need to believe in the so-called osteopathic lesions which our osteopathic colleagues seem so sure of but which they find difficult to demonstrate and prove to others.

3. Iatrogenic (*iatric*-pertaining to medicine or physicians + genesis = production) ailments are alarmingly frequent at times and in certain places, and doctors by their training have been ill prepared to deal with them. These are illnesses caused by doctor activities or their medicines. Doctors haven't yet fully understood many drugs and treatment facilities, including the antihistamines, radiation therapy, steroids, anti-cancer chemicals and some antibiotics. The scourge of doctor-caused disease has accompanied modern medical treatment like an evil talisman. I will give the result of only one study of their frequency out of many available.

A survey by Dr. E. M. Schimmel, chief resident at Yale-New Haven Hospital, published in the *Annals of Internal Medicine,* about ten years ago is now an historical document. An eight-month study in a hospital connected with the Yale University School of Medicine, revealed a virtual epidemic of iatrogenic disease: "Of 1014 patients there were 240 iatrogenic episodes occurring in 198 of the patients. Twenty per cent of the patients at risk suffered one or more episodes of medical complications in the hospital—it caused or contributed significantly to more than one in ten of all the hospital deaths."

Sixteen deaths were related to what the researcher refers to as noxious episodes. "Of the 240 iatrogenic episodes 48 were graded major, 82 moderate and 110 minor, and 105 persisted after discharge from hospital."

Iatrogenic disease constitutes a peculiarly difficult problem for doctors. They are learning about the virtues and dangers of new drugs and therapies as fast as they can, but it is a slow process. For instance, digitalis is a life-saving drug for many types of heart disease, but it took physcians of many countries working together five or six decades to learn under what precise conditions it was helpful and when it could be lethal for those same heart patients. In my own experience I lived through the earliest period of penicillin therapy and recall that we saw no allergic reactions to its use until about five years after its introduction.

4. There has been insufficient emphasis on prevention of disease and health maintenance plans. The history of medicine shows that few, if any, diseases have been controlled by treatment alone. On the other hand, many have been mastered by preventive measures. Today our approach to many killers of mankind such as heart disease, arteriosclerotic disease and arthritis contains a very slim content of preventive knowledge. In truth, medicine after hundreds of years has not come to grips with personal hygiene but is still dealing with therapeutic measures.

5. More attention needs to be given to the age-old problem of abortion. What is a workable legal basis for therapeutic abortion by practicing doctors? Are there precise major health

conditions on which we can agree in making abortion permissible?

6. More attention too should be given to the use of "the pill" and family planning. How much responsibility should the practicing physician accept for disseminating advice?

7. And, finally, student doctors planning careers as general practitioners need more instruction in the care of the elderly and senile, with emphasis on the progress being made in this area.

As the image of the general practitioner declined, for real or fancied reasons, and fewer young men were choosing to follow in his footsteps, he became a most controversial figure and the subject of innumerable articles asserting that he was obsolescent, on the one hand, and on the other that there was vital need for him in the modern social set-up. During these same years of controversy and criticism (1930's through the 1950's) numerous surveys of general practice in medical care showed clearly that most people thought their own family physician was satisfactory. They judged him to be a good doctor. Their criticism of doctors as a whole was based largely on their suspicions of the aims and activities of medical associations. This seemed trustworthy evidence that medical organizations were getting farther away from people.

Before my eleven-year stint (1954-1965) as executive director of the fledgling College of General Practice of Canada, I was a member of the board of directors of the Ontario Medical Association for five years, and president in 1949-50. Also, I sat for three years on the council of the Canadian Medical Association, its governing body. I say these things in order to add that during these years I had considerable experience with medical organizations and the result was that I became skeptical of their ability to give adequate leadership to doctors in active practice, especially to general practitioners. It was discouraging to realize, as I did after a time, that little effective help could be expected from medical associations with respect to problems of private medical practice.

The Canadian Medical Association has done much magnificent work in developing various health services. It founded the Royal College of Physicians and Surgeons, the College of Family Physicians of Canada and the Canadian Hospital Accreditation Association. But it never did play much part in the operational aspects of medical practice, or show interest really in the problems of general practitioners. The Canadian Medical Association (C.M.A.) is something like a holding company under the peculiar set-up of the British North America Act. It deals with broad health policies rather than with the details of medical practice. For these and other reasons the C.M.A. appeared to some to be more concerned with protecting its vested interests than with promoting the health of Canadian people.

Reluctantly I came to feel that the powers-that-be in professional medicine were trying to ease the general practitioner out while at the same time they were singing his praises. Certainly many in prominent places believed that the only good medicine was specialist medicine. I concluded that the collective well-being of doctors as revealed by their association activities could never equal the social value of private competence, the good work being done by a multitude of honest, capable physicians quietly pursuing their vocation in cities and hamlets across the country. It would be a pity if the one displaced the other. I became convinced that the medical profession would be saved not by its organizations but by the sum total of the common sense and humanity of its individual practicing members.

Medical organization must learn to trust general practitioners. And why not? They are the doctors closest to people. They heal more of the broken-hearted, repair more of the injured and deprived, and live with the poor and dying who are without influence and hope. Adaptation is the juice of family medicine —the G.P. adapts to the needs of people or closes up shop.

The first important move toward the renaissance of the general practitioner occurred in 1954. That was a red-letter year for him when some four hundred general practitioners from across Canada combined to organize a national college of general practice. The Canadian Medical Association assisted by sponsoring it and donating $10,000 to start it off. This college has been so successful that there is now no fear that general practice will perish in the foreseeable future. The personalized services of the general practitioner are not to be replaced soon by a battery of experts in surgery, psychiatry, medicine, etcetera. The future problem of the college is to assure that it maintains its proper stature. These are all reasonable assumptions.

The doctors involved in this pioneering venture decided to stake their hopes on an educational approach. They believed that the only sure way for general practice to survive was through better education which could put the family physician on a firm academic and clinical basis with his specialist colleagues. Their extensive program aimed at three things:

1. A more realistic training in medical school for the practice of general medicine, with senior general practitioners on the teaching staff. For this it was necessary to have the aid of medical schools, and fortunately their cooperation was promptly given.

2. Two or three years' internship training for general practice after finishing medical school, with the idea of making preparation for general practice as long and arduous as internship training for the specialties. This was based on the conviction that the brightest young men and women in the medical school are attracted to the difficult. In fact, the College of General Practice aimed at making general practice a specialty of its own and it would be one of the most difficult specialties.

3. Through a continuing upgrading program of study they would try to prevent the professional obsolescence of practicing general physicians. With education from graduation to the grave, "the family doctor would never be through learning." The College started off by boldly declaring that continuing membership in it was dependent upon the submission of evidence every two years of 100-hours' refresher-course study. This

required the establishment of refresher courses and post-graduate facilities across Canada so that family doctors wherever they lived could meet the study requirements without too much sacrifice.

The College was the only professional body in Canada with regulations to keep its members abreast of progress. The founders weren't fooling. This condition of membership cost the College many members in the early years, but eventually it proved its worth. Many specialist colleagues, educators, and hospital authorities in time were convinced that the College was serious in its efforts to keep general practitioners alert to what was going on in medicine and, best of all, members of the College themselves found that refresher courses made general practice more interesting and more satisfying.

Stimulated by the success of their college and its program, Canadian general practitioners are now calling themselves "family physicians." This is much more than a mere change of name. As never before, they are probing the dynamics of the family, the natural unit of our society. Many specialists are aiding family doctors in this. Psychiatrists too, for instance, have discovered the family and some have abandoned the long and wearisome psychoanalysis technique in favor of a more realistic active family therapy, as exemplified by the teachings of Dr. Nathan B. Epstein of the Family Practice Unit of McMaster University in Hamilton, Ontario.

Family medicine defines the service the *family physician* is specifically trained to provide. It is that body of medicine that encompasses the five major clinical disciplines: surgery, pediatrics, psychiatry, and obstetrics and gynecology, together with the social and behavioral sciences as they influence health and disease. *Family practice* is the application of this body of knowledge to the needs of the community.

The College in its earliest days as a college of general practice found it impossible to define general practice in realistic terms for purposes of teaching. In shifting emphasis to the general practitioner-family doctor concept, the College finds the above definition of family medicine a valued guide in its efforts to produce community doctors of professional competence and human understanding. For the end product in training for family medicine is a type of doctor skillful in his personal relationships with patients and as a diagnostician of human ailments.

The College of General Practice under its new name of The College of Family Physicians of Canada has made very satisfying progress. There are now five full-time professors of family medicine in our medical schools at Calgary, London, Hamilton, Halifax and Toronto; and in universities and medical schools all over Canada formal departments or divisions of family medicine have been set up, teaching units for graduates and undergraduates established, and internship or residency training programs put into operation.

In 1970 there was a marked increase in the number of medical students on graduation choosing family medicine as a career in all Canadian medical schools teaching family medicine, with one or two exceptions. In Dalhousie Medical School, one of the earliest in this field, more than 70 per cent of its graduates in 1970 chose family medicine and in 1971 the figure was more than 90 per cent. This is encouraging though it is too early for a long-term assessment. It is significant too that of the 300 candidates who sat for certification examinations in 1971, 270 were practicing doctors—indicating that certification in family medicine is appealing to many experienced general practitioners

This certification in family medicine is open to two categories of candidates: those who have emerged from the recognized internship and residency training programs following medical school graduation; and those physicians who have been in general practice at least five years and have been either active members of the College of Family Physicians during that time or can demonstrate at least 250 hours of approved post-graduate studies.

Dr. Donald I. Rice, Executive Director of the College of Family Physicians, asserts that young people today have a greater social consciousness and a greater awareness of people's needs than ever before, and he feels that this may be a reason why medical graduates of today choose family medicine rather than the traditional specialties.

The general practitioner-family doctor does not need to be as overworked as he is—or so his College is beginning to believe. The College acknowledges that other health workers can provide much health care, as demonstrated by the McMaster University Department of Family Care in Hamilton. Here it is being proved that the nurse practitioner, properly trained and working with the family doctor at the ambulatory care level, can perform many of the traditional duties of the doctor, thereby leaving him free to deal with problems that require his particular training and experience.

This is something I have long believed—that nurses can do more medical work than they have in the past and do it better because they have more time. I am convinced of this because of my own experience with a succession of competent and dedicated nurses—like Lena Robinson, my first office nurse, Annie Johnston, who was capable of assisting in major surgery in the home, and the veteran MacQuaig sisters, Agnes and Cora. The latter had served with the armed forces in World War I and returned to work for a few years in Michael Reese Hospital in Chicago, one of the best equipped hospitals in the world. When later they returned to their home town to live more leisurely, it was my good fortune—and my patients'—that I found them always available for full-time service to the seriously ill. And by full time I mean a twelve-hour day. Nurses like these can be entrusted with countless time-consuming chores. They can accompany a doctor on some of his house calls, such as initial visits to ailing elderly patients, and then follow up by making subsequent visits alone. I know this is heresy to some of my colleagues, but it will not always be so.

Medical group practice, in Canada as elsewhere, is a recent development of major significance. More and more doctors are finding some form of group effort advantageous. A committee of the Canadian Medical Association, of which Dr. E. K. Lyon of

Leamington, Ontario, was chairman, in 1967 published a report about group practices in Canada and in it defined a group as consisting "of at least three duly registered practitioners of medicine who practice together from a common office, sharing common records, pooling professional income and distributing earnings on a pre-arranged basis." Such professional teamwork has grown in popularity over the years. Whereas about 6 per cent of Canadian doctors worked in groups during the 1920's, by the 1950's figures showed a rise to 45 per cent.

Partnerships of two doctors have also increased greatly in number. And it has become common practice for neighboring doctors to cover for each other on certain evenings, holidays and week-ends.

The CMA report states: "Probably the basic underlying reason for the emergence of 'grouped' medicine is as a counter-balance to the division of medicine into more specialties with a separate specialty for almost every organ of the body." This is a view with which I take some issue. I believe the chief reason for the blossoming of group medicine is that it serves the doctors themselves as a defense against the burgeoning demand for services. The emphasis today is on health and a group interposes itself between the doctors and this public demand, which seems unlimited.

But at the core of medical practice the patient remains—an individual with intangible qualities, all of which are medicine's concern. A patient cannot take his liver only or his heart only to his doctor. The whole man goes, including his deafness, his ingrown toe nails and his worries. A group can give wider coverage to any symptom or complaint than a single physician can. It is yet to be proved, however, whether group medicine is more efficient than solo medicine.

To mention another interesting development in the widening activity of today's doctors, many of them are leaving well-established practices to go to developing countries to help set up hospitals and medical schools, and even to instruct the physicians there. Men who come to mind include Dr. E. Kirk Lyon of

Leamington, serving a period as a general surgeon in the Caribbean; Dr. Roger Whitman of Seaforth, who was in Kenya; and my son-in-law, Dr. John Mowbray, an internist of Saskatoon, who went first to Afghanistan and then to steaming-hot mid-Java—and will not thank me for mentioning him here. Some two hundred Canadian physicians were so employed abroad in 1970, their activities auguring well for an improved Canadian doctor image in the world.

In so many ways the evolution of the traditional general practitioner into a modern family doctor is bringing more science to the art of medicine. Research into family life is already yielding an amazing amount of helpful new information. Witness how family doctors are now discussing realistically and sensibly such questions as masturbation, sexual maturity and sexual pathology in marriage. This is in marked contrast to my student days when instruction on sexuality went little beyond the anatomy of the sex organs. The study of the family is an excellent base from which to give community doctors more expertise in every-day psychiatry and preventive medicine. It can instruct us about abortion, family planning and the care of the elderly and senile. In fact, one doesn't have to be a very perceptive seer to predict that there is opening up a whole new world with a battery of aids to enable the family to function better.

The College of Family Physicians with its many units can take some credit for healthy new attitudes that are everywhere apparent. Doctors are showing to-day more humanity. They are talking more about the human aspects of people's needs, their emotional problems. The profession is realizing more clearly how much of medicine is the science of feelings rather than the science of physical ailments. . . . People are expecting fuller explanations of their ailments and refusing to accept less. This is wholesome and no threat to doctors. . . . People are more willing to go through extensive technical investigations if guided by considerate physicians. . . . It is becoming more apparent that a division between private and public health is inadvisable, that we cannot chop up health into housing, welfare, church and school components. . . . Even governments are listening more to the personal complaints and wailings of people. Note the anti-cigarette advertising legislation by our Liberal Ottawa government and the Parcost program of the Ontario government for the easement of high drug costs and retention of quality control. The latter may be far from an effective measure but at least it is a move to aid the people in getting lower drug bills. . . . Best of all, a fresh wind of social consciousness and humanity has been blowing through the councils of the venerable Canadian Medical Association since the mid-1960's. They have ceased to waffle on some of the social problems involving medicine, as witness their recent actions on such matters as abortion legislation, the non-medical use of drugs and venereal disease control.

Specific efforts to improve community medical care are coming fast. For instance, 1. Dr. J. T. Colquhoun, President of the Ontario Medical Association in 1972, wrote to all the Association members asking them to give thought to what is perhaps the major problem of G.P.'s public relations, namely, their after-hours and emergency coverage. . . . 2. The serious deficiencies in training programs that neglected to instruct family doctors in psychiatry and musculo-skeletal disorders are being remedied. . . . 3. Old problems like abortion, family planning and the care of the elderly and senile are receiving much more attention.

Some critics suggest that in five years the superior-trained family doctors may become disenchanted and leave the field. If this tendency develops, then it is the task of the College of Family Physicians to keep their fields attractive. Another criticism is that the creation of certified family doctors creates an élite group with an unwholesome division of G.P.s into the good and the not-so-good. This argument has never impressed me. If the not-so-good doctor becomes fearful of his better-trained brother, he can voluntarily choose to join the good. There is no compulsion to be or remain in either group. But, most important, if this élitism brings better medicine to communities it needs no further justification.

We can realistically conclude that the Canadian G.P. is alive, vigorous and exuberant as a result of having shifted his aspirations to become a people's doctor, a general practitioner-family doctor physician. The same thing is happening to our American colleagues south of the border. The response to this new approach has been encouraging and even exhilarating. Governments have firmly supported the idea of medicine being geared to communities. Medical schools have committed themselves with bricks and mortar, personnel and money and are assuming some responsibility for the competence of family doctors in their geographic areas. And, most happily, there has been no lack of dedicated senior practitioners in all provinces to give wise leadership to the College of Family Physicians: Drs. John Corley of Calgary, Andrew Hunter of London and Pierre Houle of Trois Rivières are a few out of many. There is no reason to doubt that talented senior men will continue to come forward as leaders.

Superbly talented individuals in any professional field are rare, but every generation produces a few of them. Let me introduce you briefly to the wisest physician it has been my privilege to know. He was born twenty miles from my home town, near the village of Teeswater. On graduating from the early McKillop Veterinarian College in Toronto about the beginning of this century, he became one of its teachers, then went on to do a stint of two years as a veterinarian surgeon in the Philippines in the Spanish-American War. Following that, he entered Northwestern Medical School in Chicago, graduated and settled down as a general practitioner on Lincoln Avenue, Chicago, a staff member of the Swedish Covenant Hospital. His name was Dr. Duncan Mackenzie, the only Mackenzie listed in the huge Chicago telephone directory.

I met him this way. The editor of our local newspaper became ill with arthritis and weakness so severe he was confined to bed. I feared he was dying. One summer afternoon a tall thin elderly man entered my office wholly unannounced and introduced himself:

"I am the editor's doctor brother from Chicago. Don't be alarmed. I am here to help him and to help you. I will live with my brother for a week and then come in and tell you all I know about his sickness."

One week later he gravely announced: "I don't know what is the matter with my brother, but he will not get better. In a couple of months his wife will ask for a consultant from Toronto. Bring someone who has a special knowledge of arthritis and who will probably recommend one of the newer vaccines. Try them, but they will be of no avail. I will not be back. Just be kind to him. I will be grateful if you will watch him closely for some signs and symptoms that will give us a clue to what ails him. After he is gone, write to me what you have observed."

Dr. Mackenzie's predictions could not have been more accurate. I reported my progress observations to him as he had requested, and after a delay of six months or so he replied that his brother quite possibly had Hodgkin's disease of the mediastinum, a low-grade cancer of the glands of the chest.

Thereafter Dr. Mackenzie spent many of his summer vacations in my area near his childhood home. For a couple of weeks each summer for some ten years he would accompany me on my visits to patients, provided I never, never asked him for any comments in the presence of the sick or their relatives. He was a remarkably keen observer of people; their appearance, their speech, and even the order in which they reported their symptoms had a significance for him. In his examinations he was gentleness itself. He always insisted that he had learned much from his training as a veterinarian. "My patients, the animals, could not talk to me and I had to depend largely upon my five senses in treating them."

His skill in observation was uncanny. I owe much to his teaching of how to look, listen and then try to draw one's own conclusions. On one occasion it took him scarcely a moment to diagnose diabetes solely from the odor in the patient's bedroom.

Another time, after watching me interview a patient, he casually remarked, "That man has some kidney trouble along with his other troubles."

"How do you know?" I asked.

"The sheen of his eyes gives him away."

He would try to estimate precisely the age of an old person by noting the degree of wasting of the temporal muscles in the temporal fossae of the side of the skull just back of the forehead. All doctors have seen elderly folk where this wasting is extreme, even to a falling away of the temple regions. Dr. Mackenzie was constantly challenging me to go as far as possible in diagnosing the condition of people from my own observations and from listening to them. He had a wealth of information about people in health and disease gleaned from a life-time's study of the effects of ageing, rest, exercise and various foods.

You will note that he did not come back to see his brother after his initial visit, when he had deliberately bid him good-bye forever. Don't deduce from this that he was cold and unfeeling. Years later when he learned that his wife had incurable cancer, he immediately gave her his whole attention; he locked his office door, to unlock it again after her funeral one and a half years later.

Duncan Mackenzie was one of the rare breed.

As for me, I have no nostalgia for my years of practice, whether solo or with an associate. But though I worked from a position of strength—one of trust by my people—there were too many gaps in our knowledge of family care. It is thrilling to see some of these gaps being filled so soon with newer scientific and administrative tools. May the younger doctors coming on remember something of the old traditions of service cherished by the best of their predecessors.

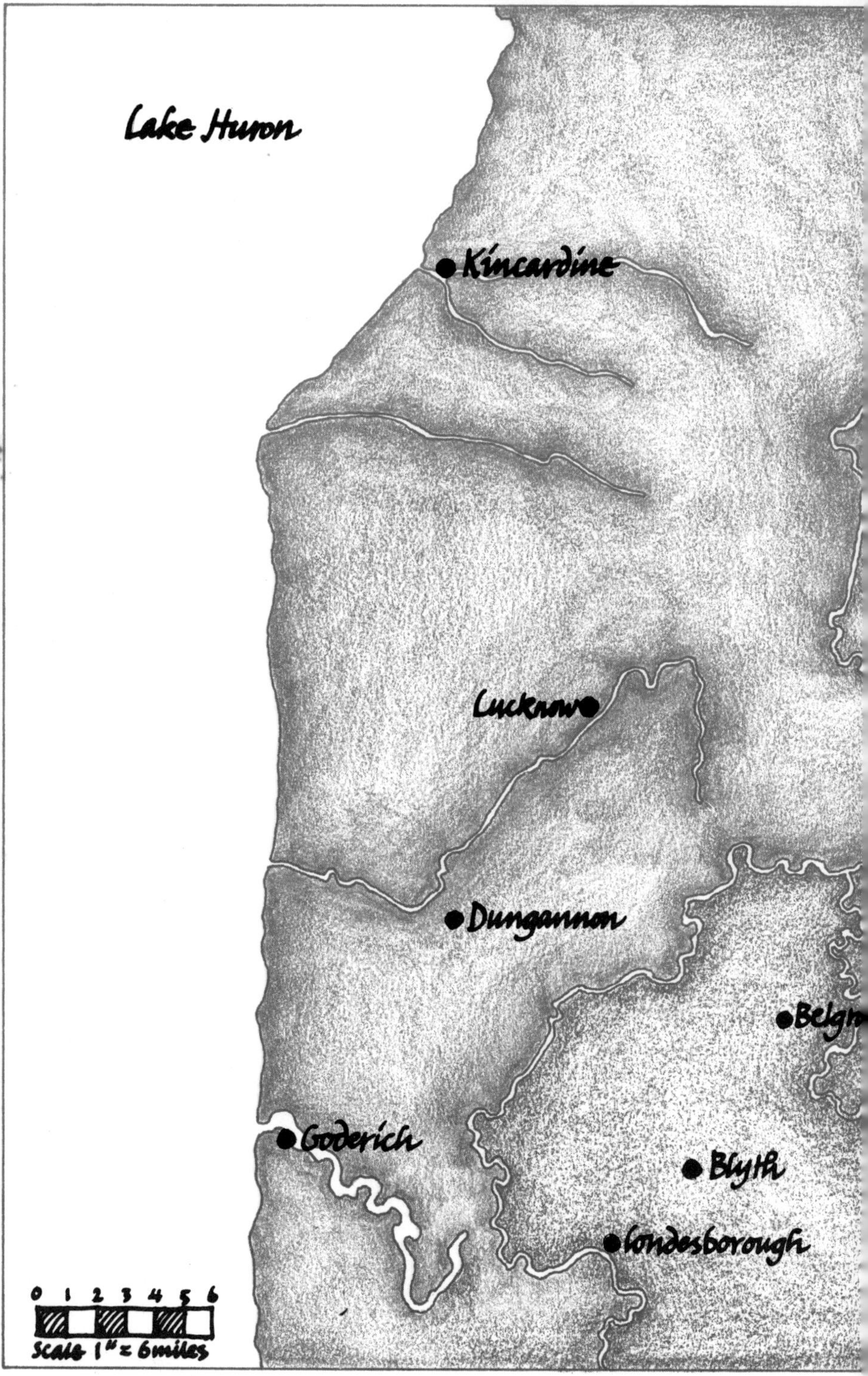
Lake Huron
Kincardine
Lucknow
Dungannon
Goderich
Blyth
Londesborough
0 1 2 3 4 5 6
Scale 1" = 6miles